Synthesis Lectures on Learning, Networks, and Algorithms

Series Editor

Lei Ying, ECE, University of Michigan–Ann Arbor, Ann Arbor, USA

The series publishes short books on the design, analysis, and management of complex networked systems using tools from control, communications, learning, optimization, and stochastic analysis. Each Lecture is a self-contained presentation of one topic by a leading expert. The topics include learning, networks, and algorithms, and cover a broad spectrum of applications to networked systems including communication networks, data-center networks, social, and transportation networks.

James Hughes · Sheridan Houghten ·
Michael Dubé · Daniel Ashlock ·
Joseph Alexander Brown · Wendy Ashlock ·
Matthew Stoodley

AI Versus Epidemics

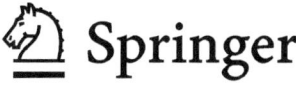

Springer

James Hughes
St. Francis Xavier University
Antigonish, NS, Canada

Michael Dubé
University of Guelph
Guelph, ON, Canada

Joseph Alexander Brown
Department of Computing Science
Thompson Rivers University
Kamloops, BC, Canada

Matthew Stoodley
Department of Mathematics and Statistics
University of Guelph
Guelph, ON, Canada

Sheridan Houghten
Department of Computer Science
Brock University
St. Catharines, ON, Canada

Daniel Ashlock
University of Guelph
Guelph, ON, Canada

Wendy Ashlock
Guelph, ON, Canada

ISSN 2690-4306   ISSN 2690-4314 (electronic)
Synthesis Lectures on Learning, Networks, and Algorithms
ISBN 978-3-031-64372-9   ISBN 978-3-031-64373-6 (eBook)
https://doi.org/10.1007/978-3-031-64373-6

This Springer imprint is published by the registered company Springer Nature Switzerland AG
The registered company address is: Gewerbestrasse 11, 6330 Cham, Switzerland

If disposing of this product, please recycle the paper.

Preface

At the beginning of the COVID-19 pandemic, the authors of this book formed a research group that met weekly to discuss how we could apply our research to the public health emergency. The group includes mathematicians, computer scientists, and bioinformaticians. We have expertise in computational intelligence including evolutionary algorithms, genetic programming, and agent-based modelling and in combinatorial graph theory. We all worked though the pandemic, moving our minds from our normal diverse tasks. We were compelled by the moment to work on this problem. Given the severity of the problem, we felt a responsibility to use and develop technologies to enable and inform the most effective and least disruptive solutions. Besides doing this research, we took on our roles as educators, many of us speaking locally on vaccine deployment and public health topics.

Our first idea was that when (and if) vaccines were developed they were likely to be in short supply. So, we started by developing a "smart" system for vaccine deployment that would minimize the spread of the virus with the fewest possible vaccines. The system would be based on an agent-based model of the spread of the epidemic in combinatorial graphs representing contact networks. Along the way, we developed techniques for creating models of contact networks from the public data released on the number of cases each day and also techniques for visualizing and interpreting results on very large graphs.

In the event that vaccines were developed, our communities chose to use a much simpler algorithm for deployment—give the vaccine first to the people most at risk. This was a reasonable decision, and we do not fault the hard-working public health decision makers. Our hope is that the tools in this book will help with making plans for the next epidemic, possibly limiting the need for lockdowns or allowing for smarter lockdowns. The tools developed are also useful for solving other problems. For people working on those problems, we hope that this book provides a helpful example of how our techniques can be applied.

We sadly lost Daniel Ashlock while this book was being written. His last public lecture in 2021 was talking about the Russian Sputnik V vaccine at a meeting of a

Western-focused university in Kazan, debunking the various claims about 5G networks, government tracking, and sterilization. He was responsible for a number of people "on the fence" getting inoculated, including a few who would later be diagnosed with COVID and survive. Till the end he was selfless and trying to save lives, even as his own was nearing the end. This book has been completed in his memory and in the hope that his work will continue to inspire students to use their knowledge to help others.

Antigonish, Canada   James Hughes
St. Catharines, Canada   Sheridan Houghten
Guelph, ON, Canada   Michael Dubé
Guelph, Canada   Matthew Stoodley
Guelph, Canada   Daniel Ashlock
Niagara-on-the-Lake, Canada   Joseph Alexander Brown
Guelph, Canada   Wendy Ashlock
August 2022

Acknowledgments

This research was supported in part by ResearchNS' Nova Scotia COVID-19 Health Coalition, consisting of Dalhousie University, Dalhousie University Medical Research Foundation, QEII Health Science Centre Foundation, IWK Foundation, Dartmouth General Hospital Foundation, Nova Scotia Health Authority, and Research Nova Scotia.

This research was also supported in part by the Natural Sciences and Engineering Research Council of Canada (NSERC).

This research was enabled in part by support provided by Compute Ontario (www.computeontario.ca), ACENET (www.ace-net.ca/), and Compute Canada (www.computecanada.ca).

This research was also supported in part by the Heaps Chair Endowment Fund at St. Francis Xavier University through the Dr. H. Stanley and Doreen Alley Heaps Chairship, which promotes the constructive interaction of computer science with liberal arts, such as language and communication, ethics, philosophy, political science, and social history.

August 2022

James Hughes
Sheridan Houghten
Michael Dubé
Matthew Stoodley
Daniel Ashlock
Joseph Alexander Brown
Wendy Ashlock

Contents

Introduction

At the end of 2019, the world was subjected to a terrible pandemic. Not only was there a death toll of millions from the pandemic itself, but people lost jobs, businesses, and livelihoods from the emergency measures taken to curb the pandemic. In addition, mental illness increased due to fear and the constant feeling of alienation over lock-downs and lack of communal events. The education of children was severely damaged by the move to online schooling.

The pandemic has contributed directly or indirectly to destabilization of a number of global governments, the creation of protest movements, and even has been a contributing factor to the end of the post cold war stabilization of the former Soviet Union and actions by the People's Republic of China to exert control on Hong Kong and the Republic of China. It has been used as a control method in several totalitarian nations. It has seriously stifled efforts at liberalization and globalization of the economies, through the reduction in logistical supply chains, international travel, and business development/capitalization.

It caused a sharp increase in the "fear index"—the Chicago Board Options Exchange maintains the ticker symbol of VIX which measures the volatility in options on the S&P 500. This volatility is a surrogate for the uncertainty of the future economy. The index since the inception of its tracking has two major peaks, the first in late 2008, coinciding with the U.S. subprime mortgage crisis and global financial crisis of 2008, and the second in March 2020, as the pandemic was in the "first wave."

The economic, political, and health effects may never be fully known or accounted for. The impacts of this pandemic have caused a number of knock-on effects as opportunities lost are rarely well understood. What would the business have been like if it did not have to lockdown? What surgeries would have been done if the hospital bed was open? What job would they have if the company did not have a layoff? Who would have been elected and

J. Hughes et al., *AI Versus Epidemics*, Synthesis Lectures on Learning, Networks, and Algorithms, https://doi.org/10.1007/978-3-031-64373-6_1

what would have been their policy if they had not have had a pandemic? At some point, these are no longer questions which can be reasonably asked by economists, scientists, political scientists, or historians, but become the realm of alternative history science fiction and fantasy writers. A question more for *The Man in the High Castle* than *The Ivory Tower*.

Yet, humanity has faced such issues in the past. For example, the great black death of 1346 (bubonic plague), the smallpox reaching the Americas in 1721, or the flu pandemic of 1918 (H1N1 influenza A). These pandemics formed an indelible mark on society. But, they have not led to the apocalyptic doomsday, and in each of these stories there have been tales of not just the trials of those involved, but in the advances of those who fought back. Much like Dr. Rieu from Albert Camus' *La Peste*, we are left with the outcome of watching the gates open, and trying to find something more to love than despise in humanity.

One lesson learned is that we need to better utilize the tools available in the information technology sphere. Even with a rapidly connected and communicating world, there were failures at a number of levels to monitor, contain, and control the spread of the virus. From the initial lack of external lock-downs in China as local governments with increasing case numbers still allowed for international travel, to the poor governmental reporting of cases, which put the emphasis on business as usual, rather than ensuring health, to the mediocre preparation for the distribution, transportation, and deployment of ventilators, and finally the early days of the vaccine which led to entire third party communities building IT infrastructure systems based on crowd-sourced information when the government information systems failed. Many of these problems were issues in data collection, cleaning, and deployment.

We address possible improved responses to a number of these problems in this book. Our goal is not to chide or criticize the public health response to COVID-19; the aim of this book is to improve the set of tools available to fight the next pandemic. In addition, this is an explanation of how to use techniques of graph theory, evolutionary algorithms, and distribution over networks for problems that are not necessarily pandemic-related. The idea of this virus is a starting point, a shared experience, that we can use to talk about complex algorithms with a less abstract application.

1.1   Overview of Concepts

The algorithms and tools presented in this book are designed to model and extract information from *personal contact networks*, which represent which individuals in a population are physically in contact with one another. In the context of an epidemic, infections are passed between individuals when they are in physical proximity. As such, modelling the personal contact network is key to understanding the dynamics of an epidemic, and to managing issues arising from the epidemic.

Personal contact networks are *combinatorial graphs*, in which the *nodes* of the graph represent the individuals in the population and the *edges* represent physical connections. In fact, throughout the remainder of this book we use the terms *network* and *graph* interchangeably. Although it is assumed that most readers will have a basic understanding of graph theory, an overview is provided in Appendix A. Readers who require a more detailed introduction may consider referring to a graph theory reference book such as West (1996).

An *epidemic model* is a means of modelling the transmission of infection across the population. Many models exist that have their basis in the *SIR model*, first presented in 1927 (Kermack and McKendrick 1927). In this model, the population is separated into three non-intersecting groups: *susceptible* (those susceptible to the infection), *infected* (those currently infected) and *removed* (those who cannot be infected). Traditionally, differential equations are used with this framework to model the spread of the disease. In this book, as we are using personal contact networks, each node is given a label to indicate their current status, and this status can change as the epidemic spreads (e.g., susceptible to infected). The different models used, and the processes followed, are further described in each chapter.

1.2   Organization of the Book

The remaining chapters of this book are organized as follows.

Evolutionary computation, a methodology from within artificial intelligence, is the key underpinning for all of the algorithms and tools presented in this book. This is introduced in Chap. 2.

Several issues arise when representing a given population, such as a city or set of connected cities, as a personal contact network. The most serious of these is the sheer size of this network, while noisy data is also a significant concern. To manage these issues, *graph compression* is a useful tool, described in Chap. 3.

Often it is the case that we wish to find personal contact networks likely to result in given epidemic behaviour, such as maximizing or minimizing the total number of infections or length of the epidemic, or to best match a given "curve" of infections per day. To do so, the process of *network induction* is used, described in Chap. 4.

In the case that there is a shortage in the supply of available vaccines, governments must decide upon an order in which the individuals in the population should be inoculated, so as to minimize the effects of the epidemic. Such decisions are greatly dependent on the structure of the personal contact network. In Chap. 5, genetic programming is used to develop suitable *vaccination strategies*.

When applying the algorithms for network induction to real data, several considerations must be taken into account, most notably the size of the *search space* of possible networks. Techniques to manage these issues are presented in Chap. 6.

References

W.O. Kermack, A.G. McKendrick, A contribution to the mathematical theory of epidemics. Proc.
  R. Soc. Lond. Ser. A (Containing papers of a Mathematical and Physical Character) **115**(772),
  700–721 (1927)
D.B. West. *Introduction to Graph Theory* (Prentice Hall, Upper Saddle River, NJ, 1996)

Evolutionary Computation

2

Not a single thing within our universe evades evolution; every object, system, and idea is subject to the evolutionary process. Guided by biological, chemical, environmental, or physical constraints, human design, or the *invisible hand*, all things exist as a consequence of the evolutionary algorithm that permeates our lives. It is natural, in every sense of the word, to make use of this process in our attempts to make sense of our natural world.

This chapter provides an introduction to evolutionary computation, concentrating on Evolutionary Algorithms (EA) and Genetic Programming (GP). Both of these have the same high-level algorithm (Fig. 2.1), and much of the nuance behind the algorithms are easier to present in a more general way. Most of the differences come down to *what* we are *evolving* with our algorithms—where common EAs are generally used to evolve a solution to a problem, GP is used to evolve a *program*.

To summarize the basic idea of an EA as briefly as possible—given some problem, start with a *population* of many randomly generated solutions, *evaluate* each of them, *select* the relatively effective solutions, allow the selected individuals to exchange information and create "children", add the children to the population, and repeat over and over again for many *generations*.

Obviously the initial randomly created solutions will very likely be terrible, but over time, after hundreds, thousands, or millions of *generations*, the population is typically full of many high-quality solutions to the problem.

Throughout this chapter, the *Travelling Salesperson Problem*[1] (TSP) will be used as an example as it is one of the quintessential example problems within the field. Further, it is

---

[1] Although classically defined as the Travelling Salesman Problem, here we use salesperson.

J. Hughes et al., *AI Versus Epidemics*, Synthesis Lectures on Learning, Networks, and Algorithms, https://doi.org/10.1007/978-3-031-64373-6_2

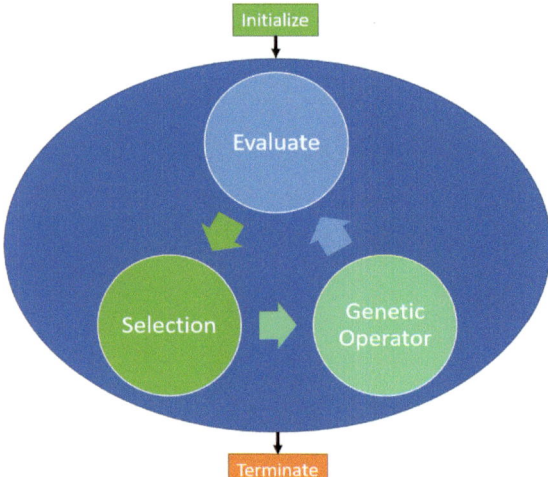

Fig. 2.1 High-level view of an evolutionary algorithm. Although there are differences in each type of evolutionary algorithm and even between individual implementations of the same algorithms, the basic idea is the same. Each starts with some form of initialization that prepares the algorithm for the evolutionary search. After initialization the main loop executes, which repeatedly evaluates the quality of each candidate solution at addressing the given problem, selects candidate solutions based on some criteria, and applies genetic operators to the selected candidate solutions. Finally, after some termination criteria is met, the algorithm halts resulting in a population of candidate solutions for the given problem

well defined, easy to understand, but is of the class NP-hard. There are many variations of the problem, and although the reader is likely familiar with the TSP, an informal definition is provided here.

Given a completely connected and undirected weighted graph, find the *Hamiltonian cycle* with the minimum total sum of edge weights along the path. The analogue to the salesperson being an individual needing to start from home, visit some number of cities, and return home while travelling as little as possible.

Bringing this back to the brief description of an EA—start with a population of randomly generated Hamiltonian cycles, evaluate each of their total path lengths, select the relatively good solutions, allow the relatively good solutions to exchange information and create new "children" Hamiltonian cycles, add the children to a population, and repeat over and over again. Again, the initial population of Hamiltonian cycles will very likely be terrible, but over time the cycles will become shorter and shorter.

2.1   Evolutionary Algorithms

The current research area of EAs is the result of the culmination of work from several individuals working on related, but different ideas. A brief history is provided here; however, this is in no way exhaustive since the field has benefited from the contributions of many as the ideas and techniques evolved.

Alan Turing highlighted, while discussing the *imitation game*,[2] the parallels between a hypothetical stochastic learning machine and the natural process of evolution (Turing 2009). His discussion included the ideas of inheriting information from parents, allowing for stochastic changes, and a selection mechanism.

In the late 1950s and early 60s multiple researchers, including Niles Barricelli from Princeton's *Institute for Advanced Research* (Barricelli 1957), started implementing these ideas to simulate evolution on a computer.

Throughout the 60s and 70s, the ideas grew in popularity and some of the popular EAs from today emerged. The idea of *Evolutionary Strategies*, a specific kind of EA, was developed by Rechenberg (1973). Lawrence Fogel et al. developed another EA called *Evolutionary Programming* (Fogel 1998, Fogel et al. 1966), and the class of EA called *Genetic Algorithms* (GAs), by far the most popular kind of EA, was developed in the 1970s by Holland (1992).

These ideas were developed independently from one another at a time when the term "evolutionary algorithm" had no real meaning. It was not until later that the generalized class of algorithms called EAs emerged based on the common core ideas among the various implementations—population based, fitness evaluation, selection, mutation, and reproduction.

There are many specific EAs, all with different strengths and weaknesses. If one generalizes further to the class of algorithms called *Evolutionary Computation* (EC), of which EAs are a subclass, one can find the popular subclass called *Swarm Intelligence* (SI). *Particle Swarm Optimization*, a popular form of SI inspired by the behaviour of flocks of birds and schools of fish, is another stochastic population based strategy with mechanisms for exchanging information between individuals.

Computational Intelligence (CI) is an even further generalization that includes algorithms such as EC, Artificial Neural Networks, and Fuzzy Logic.

One nice feature of EAs is that they are generally applicable to many problems and can obtain high quality results with little to no domain knowledge. Given the modular nature of EAs, incorporating domain knowledge is usually easy and can improve results. However, given the required computational resources and often difficult to interpret results, EAs, like most other forms of CI, are typically reserved for situations where no other strategy proves effective. For example, realistically, something like the Lin and Kernighan (1973) algorithm would be used for finding high-quality TSP solutions, but unlike specialized algorithms, the EAs are relatively trivial to implement, require minimal specialized knowledge, and in

---

[2] Commonly referred to as *The Turing Test*.

spite of this, they still produce high-quality solutions. Ultimately, however, EAs are usually reserved for difficult and complex problems when no other strategy proves effective—they are the type of algorithm you do not want to have to use.

Given how generally applicable EAs are, they have been used in countless areas within research & development and industry. Interesting examples include analog circuit synthesis (Barros et al. 2010, Rojec et al. 2019), designing restaurant layouts (Ugurlu et al. 2015), designing buildings and structures to minimize energy use (Moylan and Ross 2015, Tuhus-Dubrow and Krarti 2010), and evolutionary artwork (Secretan et al. 2008, 2011). NASA created an antenna with EAs that flew on NASA's Space Technology 5 mission (Hornby et al. 2006) and recently Uber Technologies Incorporated has been investing in the exploration of deep neuroevolution (evolving artificial neural networks) (Stanley 2018, Stanley et al. 2019). The above examples are far from exhaustive and they were chosen not for the quality of results, but for the allure and charm of the application areas.

2.1.1 Representation

As discussed above, a *population* of "candidate solutions" is evolved over many generations. A population is made up of many potential solutions to the problem at hand. How exactly a candidate solution is encoded will depend on a number of things, but a simple example can be seen in Fig. 2.2 which is depicting a bit string.

Although contrived, our goal may be to evolve a bit string to maximize its base 10 integer value. Obviously the optimal solution is a string of ones, but nevertheless, a bit string is a workable representation for the problem. In fact, bit strings were one of the early proposed representations for all problems when using EAs. The idea was that they are simple and can encode anything, as long as there was an appropriate decoding or *translation* strategy to get from the encoding to its meaning. In this example, the bit string would be the encoded base 10 number being evolved, and it is common within the field of EAs to refer to the encoded

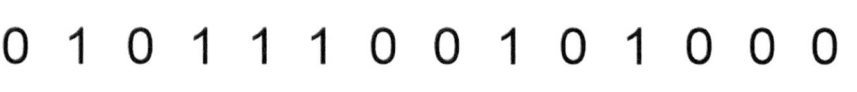

Fig. 2.2 Example of a simple bit string candidate solution. The binary values are stored in some ordered linear data structure. Although it is possible that these binary values have a direct meaning, often a bit string representation would require some decoding, or *translation* method before it could be evaluated in the context of the problem being addressed

data as a *chromosome*, and an individual chromosome would represent a point within the *genotype* space. Conversely, what the chromosome decodes to is referred to as the *candidate solution*, and they exist within the *phenotype* space.[3]

The encoding choice for a given problem has important implications for the search space and how successful the EA will be. Although this will be discussed in more detail within Sect. 2.1.2, to get an appreciation for how the encoding has an impact, consider the landscape of the search space—how one can move between the possible values. Assuming a 14 bit unsigned integer, there are a total of 2^{14}, or 16, 384 values. For any of the possible values, if we allow only the smallest possible change of adding or subtracting one to the value, there are only two adjacent values. For example, if we consider the number n, the values $n - 1$ and $n + 1$ are adjacent to n. Alternatively, when considering the encoded space, the bit string, and the smallest possible change of a bit flip, there are 14 adjacent values since any of the 14 bits may be flipped.

A bit string for maximizing a base 10 integer value would be an example of a rather *indirect* representation. If one were using a bit string for encoding TSP solutions, there would need to be a lot of decoding to translate the chromosome into a Hamiltonian cycle. An example of a more *direct* representation for TSP would be a list of numbers representing the order in which one should visit the cities—Fig. 2.3. Some amount of decoding is required, such as needing a numerical label for each city, but the encoding is much more natural for TSP when compared to a bit string.

It is usually important to ensure that the chosen encoding is able to represent all possible valid solutions; if the genotype space disallows certain points in the phenotype space, it is possible that the optimal and other high-quality solutions may be missed. However, it is also important to constrain the search space as it is much easier to explore smaller spaces. This is perhaps best explained with an example. For a TSP instance with n cities, we could represent candidate solutions with a list of length n containing integers between 0 and $(n - 1)$ representing individual cities. This encoding would allow for n^n possible points in

0 5 2 6 8 9 1 4 3 7

Fig. 2.3 Example of a more general candidate solution when compared to the bit string representation shown in Fig. 2.2. This specific example shows a permutation of 10 numbers within an ordered linear data structure. This would be an ideal representation for a problem such as the travelling salesman problem as the permutation property enforces that each city is visited once and only once. In general, however, the permutation representation is not a requirement; what exactly is stored within the candidate solution will depend on the problem and the decoding/translation method

---

[3] Although the jargon of genotype and phenotype is used here, the authors emphasize that the important take away is that the encoded and decoded information exist in separate spaces.

the genotype space. Alternatively, since a requirement for TSP is that each city is visited once and only once, one could choose to encode candidate solutions as permutations of all integers between 0 and $(n - 1)$, which would have a total of $n!$ possible points within the genotype space. Both encodings *can* encode admissible solutions, but the latter, which is far more constrained, will be a much smaller space to traverse.

2.1.2 Fitness

Each member of the population must be evaluated in order to determine how effective it is at addressing the problem at hand. The measure of a candidate solution's effectiveness is referred to as its *fitness* which is calculated with a *fitness function/measure*. Using the TSP example with the permutation encoding, a reasonable fitness measure would be the total Euclidean distance the Hamiltonian cycle requires. Given two permutations, the one with a lower total Euclidean distance would be considered better and more fit.

Along with selection (Sect. 2.1.3), the fitness values of the candidate solutions are what help guide the search. Ideally, more fit candidate solutions will have a higher likelihood to produce offspring when compared to candidate solutions with a lower fitness value. Note that the fitness value, and what is considered effective, is all relative to other candidate solutions within the population. EAs are typically used for complex problems where a known optimal is likely not known, thus an absolute measure of fitness is often not feasible.

Since the fitness values are all relative, and there is a fixed population size, there is competition for a limited set of resources. Despite this individual fitness value level thinking, it is often helpful to realize that, although changes and fitness measures are done on individual candidate solution, it is the population as a whole that is evolving.

How the fitness of a candidate solution is calculated will depend on the problem being solved. For example, with TSP, the total Euclidean distance in the Hamiltonian cycle is a reasonable choice. Assuming the ordered permutation of cities, which is a rather direct representation of the problem, there is minimal *translation/decoding* required to convert the chromosome into something that can be evaluated. Alternatively, maximizing the unsigned base 10 integer with the bit string representation requires more translation since the binary number needs to be translated into a base 10 number.

However, with the bit string example, an alternative fitness function may be used. Since we know that the optimal solution would be encoded as a bit string of all ones, instead of translating the binary number, it is possible to simply count the number of ones in the bit string—a chromosome with more ones is closer to the optimal solution even if it's base 10 integer value is less. This, however, is only possible because we have a strong understanding of the genotype (encoded candidate solution) and the phenotype spaces (what the candidate solution means). Unfortunately, in many complex real world problems, little is known about the fitness landscape and the dynamics at play within the genotype and phenotype spaces, thus it may not be possible to make similarly informed decisions.

Given the fact that EAs are generational and population based searches on rather complex problems, as one may expect, the fitness function is used many times—depending on the problem, thousands, millions, or billions of times. Most of the execution time of an EA is spent on evaluating fitness values.

2.1.3 Selection

As mentioned earlier, the mechanism for selecting which candidate solutions may reproduce and have their children added to the population plays a significant role in guiding the evolutionary search. It may be tempting to always select the top candidate solutions based on their fitness values, but this often causes the search and population to *converge* too quickly towards a local optimum—something that happens when there is a high *selection pressure*. Alternatively, randomly selecting candidate solutions irrespective of their fitness values would not be effective as we would be left with a random search—not enough selection pressure.

To hedge against premature convergence, it is desirable to have enough selection pressure to guide the search effectively, while also preserving some amount of *diversity* among the candidate solutions within the population. There are many popular strategies for selection, some of which are designed for specific EA algorithms, but a very popular and general selection strategy is *tournament selection*.

For tournament selection, one typically selects k candidate solutions randomly from the population, and from the k, the top candidate solution is selected. With this strategy, relatively fit candidate solutions are still selected, but since k will be a subset of the whole population, it ensures that some amount of diversity in the population will be preserved. Figure 2.4 shows an example of selecting a single candidate solution with a tournament size of $k = 3$. Deciding on what k value to choose will need to be determined empirically with tests, but it is not unusual to see small values chosen (2–5), even with relatively large population sizes (>100).

2.1.4 Genetic Operators

There are two categories of genetic operators—*crossover* and *mutation*. Crossover acts on two candidate solutions and provides a mechanism for transferring information between them, while mutation acts on a single candidate solution and typically makes a small change. When candidate solutions have been selected with some selection strategy, they will be copied and, before being added to the population, there is some probabilistic chance that they will undergo crossover or a mutation.

If two candidate solutions are selected for crossover, then some crossover operator will be applied to them. Like most parts of an EA there are many options to choose from for a crossover operator, but the decision will depend on the problem and representation. There

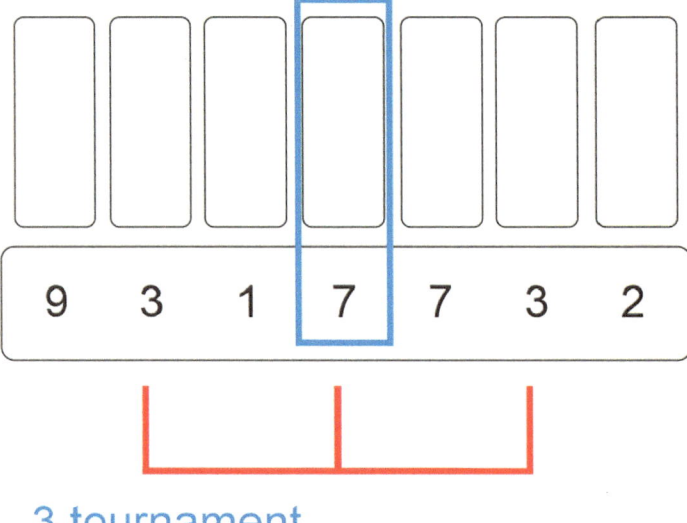

3 tournament

Fig. 2.4 Tournament selection. k candidate solutions—in this case, three—are selected at random and their fitness values are compared. The candidate solution with the best fitness of the k will be selected. This selection technique has a bias towards selecting candidate solutions with better fitness values, which is the idea, however assuming k is much smaller than the population size, it is unlikely to always be selecting the best candidate solutions within the population. This feature is important as it helps to premature convergence

are multiple reasonable crossover operators for different problems and representations. For example, a *one-point crossover*, where a single index is selected and all elements after that index are exchanged between the two candidate solutions (Fig. 2.5), would be appropriate for the bit string example. Unfortunately this crossover is not workable for the TSP example as it will very likely cause the Hamiltonian cycle to visit cities more than once while missing others. In this case, more sophisticated crossovers would be required (such as partially mapped crossover or order crossover, as depicted in Fig. 2.6). Specialized crossovers (and mutations) are also required for GP, however those are discussed in Sect. 2.1.4.

Fig. 2.5 Single-point crossover. After two candidate solutions have been selected, a single index is selected and all values following the randomly selected index are exchanged between the two candidate solutions. This crossover can be generalized to an n-point crossover where all values are exchanged between the selected indices

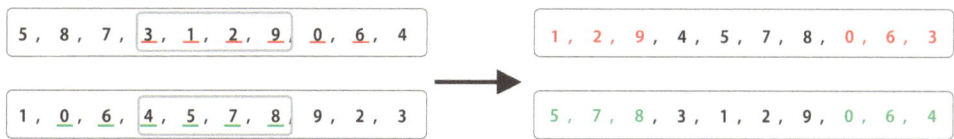

Fig. 2.6 Depiction of an ordered crossover. This crossover preserves the uniqueness of the values within the candidate solutions during crossover, which is important when working with certain representations. Although this crossover is more complex than others, the overall idea is relatively straightforward. A subset of each of the candidate solutions before crossover is chosen (indicated by the gray box on the left) and swapped between the two solutions after crossover (on the right). Then each candidate solution after crossover is filled with values that do not appear in the acquired subset in the order they appeared after the subset before crossover was applied. Consider the red values in the above example. Only the values 0, 6, 3, 1, 2, 9 are added since 4, 5, 8, and 7 are already within the candidate solution after crossover

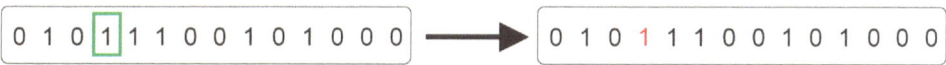

Fig. 2.7 A single point mutation on a bit string representation. Simply select an index at random and flip the bit. This mutation can be easily generalized to n-point mutation

Consider two identical bit strings. If one were to apply one-point crossover to them, no matter which index you select, the candidate solutions will not change. Crossover is the mechanism by which information is exchanged and passed to other candidate solutions, but it is not effective at adding new information to the candidate solutions—this is where mutation comes in.

Like crossover, if a candidate solution is chosen for mutation, there are many reasonable mutation operators for different problems and representations. When considering the bit string example, a reasonable choice would be a *bit flip* mutation (Fig. 2.7)—select an index in the bit string and flip the symbol at that index ($0->1$ or $1->0$). However, such a mutation would not work well for the TSP example with a permutation representation since the representation is not a bit string, and even if the mutation was generalized to simply change the city number at a given index, it would break the representation's property of containing a permutation of unique numbers. A workable alternative would be to select two indices and swap the city numbers between them.

2.2   Putting it Together

With the basic building blocks of the EAs covered, it is now simply a matter of putting them together to run the search. When referring back to Fig. 2.1, the evaluation, selection, and genetic operators are processes the are repeatedly applied to the population until stopping criteria is met.

Like most things with the EA, there is flexibility in how and when these processes are used. One common strategy is a generational application of the processes. This means the whole population is evaluated and selection is repeatedly applied to select enough chromosomes to completely fill a whole new population while probabilistically applying the genetic operators to the selected chromosomes. An alternative popular strategy is the steady state approach which does not replace a whole population, but only replaces a two chromosome at a time (two, since it is common to select two chromosomes at a time before probabilistically determining if crossover is applied).

The stopping criteria for the search will depend on the specific situation. Typically one would stop the search after some predefined number of generations/mating events have occurred, after the population's fitness has not significantly improved for some time, or once some fitness threshold is met.

Although there is no proof of convergence for a general EA, with careful tuning of the parameters and operators, the final population is often a collection of high-quality solutions for a given problem. How good the final solutions are will depend on the settings and the problem itself, but, despite no guarantees, EAs consistently produce satisfactory solutions.

2.3 Genetic Programming

Genetic programming is a specialized form of EA that ultimately has all the same core ideas and principles as most other forms of EAs developed in the latter half of the 20th century. What makes it stand out is that instead of being used to evolve solutions to a problem, GP evolves programs.[4] With this shift of objectives comes different representations and corresponding genetic operators for facilitating the evolution of programs.

The idea of GP was developed by John Koza in the late 1980s, and in the early 1990s two important books (followed by more) were written by Koza demonstrating the algorithm and its remarkable effectiveness (Koza et al. 1994, Koza 1992). Since then GP has emerged as a remarkably powerful search strategy for many types of problems.

2.4 Representation and Language

Traditionally, GP makes use of a tree structure to encode programs. Figure 2.8 depicts an example of a tree encoding for *symbolic regression*—a nonlinear form of regression analysis GP excels at. In this example, the programs being evolved are mathematical expressions, and the specific expression encoded by Fig. 2.8 is $2x + sin(x)$. Notice that in this example there are operators and operands within the nodes of the tree, and further, the operands are either constants (e.g., the number 2) or variables (e.g., the variable x). Also notice that for

---

[4] If one considers the need to find a program the *problem*, then there is even less of a distinction between GP and more general EAs.

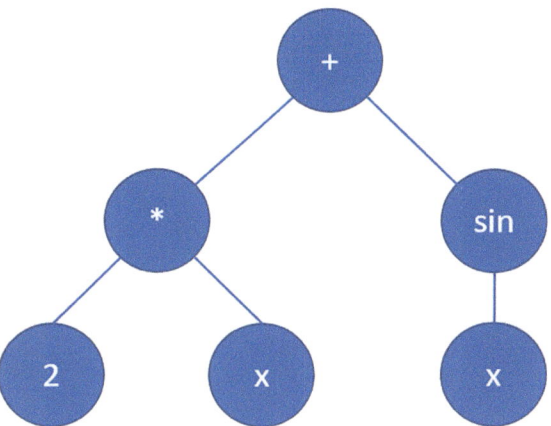

Fig. 2.8 Tree representing $2x + sin(x)$

some operators, such as addition and multiplication, require two operands, while others, like *sin*, only need one.

GP is generalizable well beyond mathematical expressions; see Fig. 2.10 for an example of a tree encoding a program representing a vaccination strategy. The set of allowed operators and operands is defined by the GP *language*, and depending on the type of problem being solved, different languages may be defined. For example, with symbolic regression, a specified set of mathematical operators and numbers will be selected; however, which operators and operands are allowed will depend on the problem (is the inclusion of trigonometric operators necessary?).

GP languages can become more complex. Consider the vaccination strategy example in Fig. 2.10. Unlike the regression example where all the operators and operands ultimately resulted in a *number*, there are multiple data types in the vaccination strategy example—numbers and Booleans.

2.5   Selection and Genetic Operators

It is common in GP to have relatively large populations when compared to other forms of EAs. As a consequence, there are specialized selection strategies to compensate for the population sizes; however, the common EA selection strategies are often still workable. The very popular tournament selection strategy with an appropriately set tournament size determined empirically through initial experiments is very common.

Like all other forms of EAs, the crossover operation must work for the encoding. With GP, since the representation is typically trees, if two candidate solutions are selected for crossover, any mechanism for exchanging information between the trees would be workable.

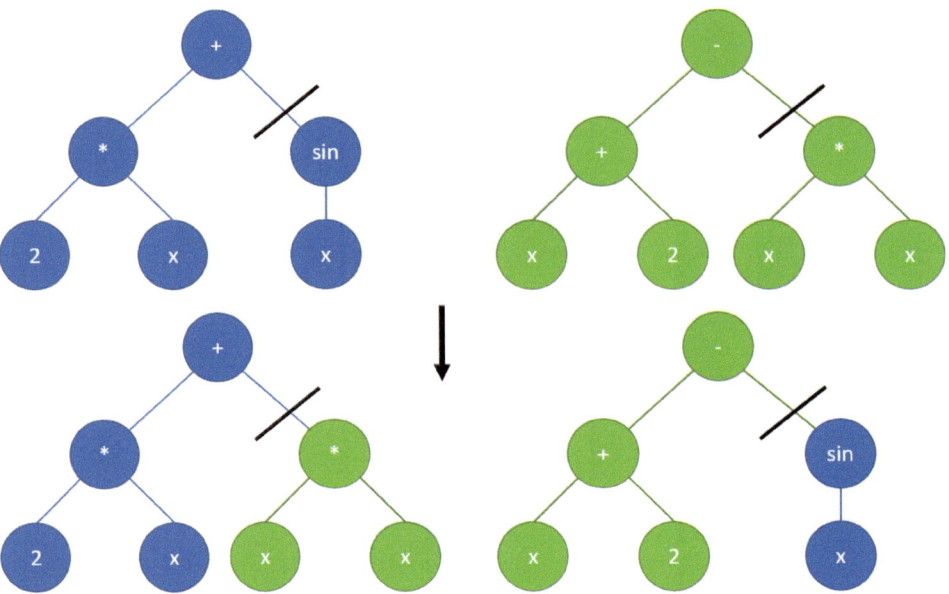

Fig. 2.9 One point crossover of subtrees

A very commonly used crossover operator is *one-point crossover*, but unlike the one-point crossover for more general EAs depicted above (Fig. 2.5), two subtrees are selected and exchanged. Figure 2.9 shows an example of one point crossover of subtrees between two mathematical expressions. This crossover may become more involved if the tree has multiple types since the return type of the subtree must match the input of the parent node, but these are manageable implementation issues.

Single point mutation is commonly used in GP—select a subtree and replace it with another randomly created subtree. The new subtree may be a single node, or a tree with multiple levels. Figure 2.12 provides a visualization of a single node subtree being replaced by a type safe single node subtree for an encoding of vaccination strategies.

Note that like most things for EAs, there are many valid and workable genetic operators for GP; GP is a very *modular* search strategy that allows the user to pick and choose their operators to fit their needs.

2.6   Genetic Programming for Vaccine Distribution

Although a detailed description of how GP is used for the purpose of discovering novel vaccination strategies for effectively slowing the spread of an infectious disease is provided in Chap. 5, a brief summary of how the ideas discussed throughout this chapter connect to the problem is presented here.

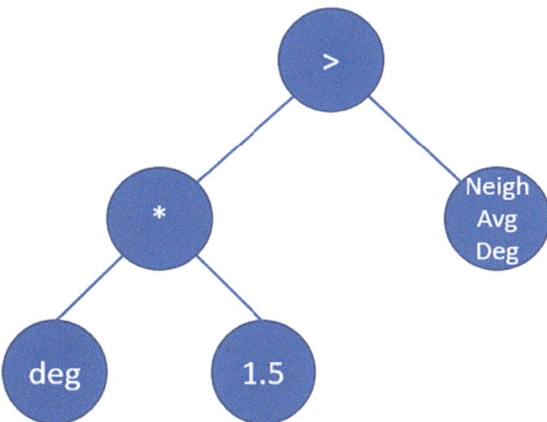

Fig. 2.10 Tree representation typical of genetic programming. In this example the internal nodes are operators and the leaf nodes are value, wither constants or parameters. This particular example is of a function/program for deciding if an individual should be vaccinated. More precisely, according to this function/program, the individual should be vaccinated if 150% of the individual's degree is greater than the average degree of their neighbours

The language for the problem includes a number of operators for numbers and Booleans, and the operands are graph measures and other *questions* about the current state of the pandemic. For example: how many individuals are currently infected?; how many infected connections does an individual have?; how many vaccines are currently available? The language is used to generate the trees representing a vaccination strategy, like the one seen in Fig. 2.10, which suggests that an individual be vaccinated if $1.5\times$ the degree of that individual is greater than the average degree of all their neighbours.

In order to evaluate the fitness of a given vaccination strategy, a full simulation of an infectious disease scenario on a graph representing a social contact network must be executed. During the simulation, individuals are vaccinated based on the encoded vaccination strategy being evaluated, which will have an impact on the spread of the disease. There are a number of reasonable measures for fitness, such as the total number of individuals that got infected during the simulation, or the maximum number of individuals infected at a given time, but the choice may depend on the goals of the user.

The selection strategy was a simple tournament selection and the genetic operators are those discussed in Sect. 2.1.4 for GP. Since the encoding has two types (numbers and Booleans), the genetic operators must be applied in a way to ensure the resulting trees are type correct. Figures 2.11 and 2.12 show examples of crossover and mutation on vaccination strategies that result in type correct trees. Notice that in both cases, since each of the points selected evaluates to a number, the replacing subtree must also evaluate to a number.

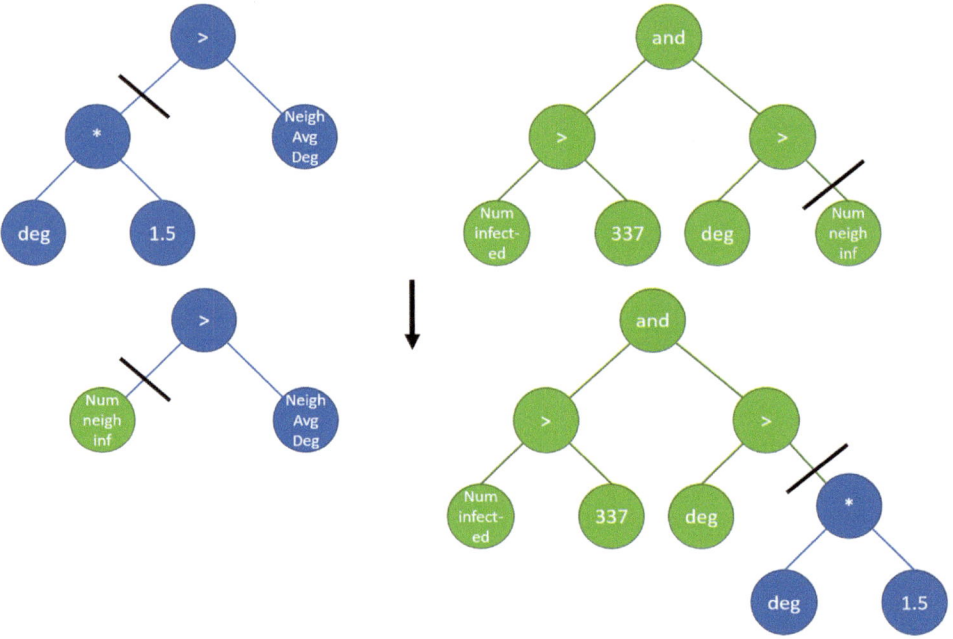

Fig. 2.11 Single point crossover on the tree representation typical of genetic programming. Simply select a node from each tree with the same return type (numerical vs. boolean in this example) and exchange the subtrees with the selected nodes as the roots between the two trees

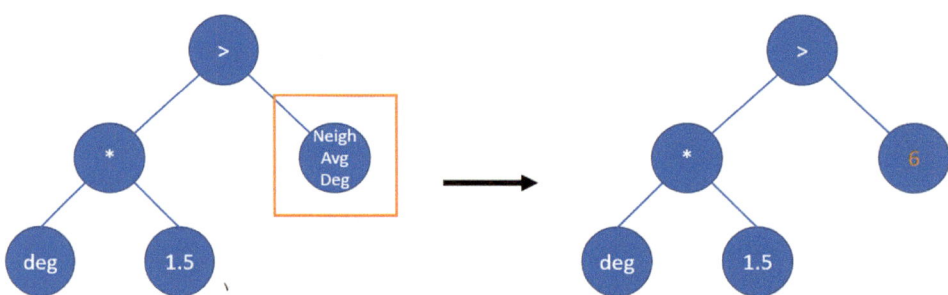

Fig. 2.12 Single point mutation for the tree representation. Simply select a single node within the tree and replace it with a randomly selected new node. If the selected node is an internal node the randomly selected new node must be an appropriate operator (taking the same number of operands and returning the correct value type). Additionally, depending on the implementation, leaf nodes may be replaced with newly generated trees

2.7   The Takeaway

The details within this chapter were deliberately kept at a high-level. Although true, this was not done because the authors feel that this level of details is sufficient for gaining an understanding of the necessary background information to follow the remained of the book. The details were kept at a high-level because EAs are intrinsically not much more than a suite of high-level ideas put together in a clever way. There may be common genetic operators and selection strategies used, but it is well accepted that there exists no silver bullet and implementing different ideas does not make an implementation any less of an EA as long as it follows the basic overarching ideas.

Remember, EAs should not always be a programmer's first choice when looking for solutions to their problems. But when push comes to shove and all else fails, they can be depended on to find quality solutions to complex problems such as the ones presented in this book.

References

N.A. Barricelli, Symbiogenetic evolution processes realized by artificial methods. Methodos **9**, 143–182 (1957)

M.F.M. Barros, J.M.C. Guilherme, N.C.G. Horta, *Analog Circuits and Systems Optimization Based on Evolutionary Computation Techniques*, vol. 9 (Springer, 2010)

D.B. Fogel, *Artificial Intelligence Through Simulated Evolution* (Wiley-IEEE Press, 1998)

L.J. Fogel, A.J. Owens, M.J. Walsh, Intelligent decision making through a simulation of evolution. Behav. Sci. **11**(4), 253–272 (1966)

J.H. Holland et al., *Adaptation in Natural and Artificial Systems: An Introductory Analysis with Applications to Biology, Control, and Artificial Intelligence* (MIT Press, 1992)

G. Hornby, A. Globus, D. Linden, J. Lohn, Automated antenna design with evolutionary algorithms, in *Space 2006* (American Institute of Aeronautics and Astronautics, 2006), pp. 7242–7249

J.R. Koza et al., *Genetic Programming II*, vol. 17 (MIT Press, Cambridge, MA, 1994)

J.R. Koza, *Genetic Programming: On the Programming of Computers by Means of Natural Selection*, vol. 1 (MIT Press, 1992)

S. Lin, B.W. Kernighan, An effective heuristic algorithm for the traveling-salesman problem. Oper. Res. **21**(2), 498–516 (1973)

K. Moylan, B.J. Ross, Interior illumination design using genetic programming, in *International Conference on Evolutionary and Biologically Inspired Music and Art* (Springer, 2015), pp. 148–160

I. Rechenberg, *Evolutionsstrategie* (Holzmann-Froboog, Stuttgart, 1973)

Ž. Rojec, Á. Bűrmen, I. Fajfar, Analog circuit topology synthesis by means of evolutionary computation. Eng. Appl. Artif. Intell. **80**, 48–65 (2019)

J. Secretan, N. Beato, D.B.D. Ambrosio, A. Rodriguez, A. Campbell, K.O. Stanley, Picbreeder: evolving pictures collaboratively online, in *Proceedings of the SIGCHI Conference on Human Factors in Computing Systems*, pp. 1759–1768 (2008)

J. Secretan, N. Beato, D.B. D'Ambrosio, A. Rodriguez, A. Campbell, J.T. Folsom-Kovarik, K.O. Stanley. Picbreeder: a case study in collaborative evolutionary exploration of design space. Evol. Comput. **19**(3), 373–403 (2011)

K.O. Stanley, Welcoming the era of deep neuroevolution (2018). https://eng.uber.com/deep-neuroevolution/

K.O. Stanley, J. Clune, J. Lehman, R. Miikkulainen, Designing neural networks through neuroevolution. Nat. Mach. Intell. **1**(1), 24–35 (2019)

D. Tuhus-Dubrow, M. Krarti, Genetic-algorithm based approach to optimize building envelope design for residential buildings. Build. Environ. **45**(7), 1574–1581 (2010)

A.M. Turing, Computing machinery and intelligence, in *Parsing the Turing Test* (Springer, 2009), pp. 23–65

C. Ugurlu, I. Chatzikonstantinou, S. Sariyildiz, M.F. Tasgetiren, Evolutionary computation for architectural design of restaurant layouts, in *2015 IEEE Congress on Evolutionary Computation (CEC)* (IEEE, 2015), pp. 2279–2286

Graph Compression

The algorithms presented in this chapter may be applied to any unweighted or weighted graphs. Concerning epidemics, they can be applied to personal contact networks. For example, contact tracing and various proximity-detecting apps can track movement and contact between individuals. Combining all this information for a large population such as a city or state would produce an extremely large graph. Ideally one would wish to analyze and determine recommendations based upon the information found in the graph, however the size and complexity of the graph makes this very difficult. Graph compression can reduce and simplify the size to make analysis more manageable. As such, it can be applied as a first step, when dealing with a large real-world network, prior to some of the other analysis carried out in the other chapters of this book. In addition, the information stored in the graph is likely to be quite noisy, with some information missing or incorrect. Compression of the graph can help to provide a "big picture" view of community structure, and to smooth out irregularities due to noise.

The compression of the personal contact network provides a classification of pockets of potential high transmission, allowing for public health groups to better target sparse resources. This also allows for a more targeted response for quarantines, social distancing rules, or other mitigation efforts, based upon a high-level view of social interactions rather than details on individuals.

© The Author(s), under exclusive license to Springer Nature Switzerland AG 2024 21
J. Hughes et al., *AI Versus Epidemics*, Synthesis Lectures on Learning,
Networks, and Algorithms, https://doi.org/10.1007/978-3-031-64373-6_3

3.1   Concepts of Graph Compression

Graph compression entails reducing the number of nodes in the graph by merging nodes into *supernodes*. Correspondingly, the edges associated with a supernode are in fact *superedges* as they can represent multiple edges: as will be seen, these edges represented by the superedge may be to, from, or between the nodes merged into the supernode.

Suppose we have a graph G with a set of vertices (or nodes) V and set of edges E. Prior to compression, the number of nodes in the graph is $N_o = |V|$ and the number of edges in the graph is $E_o = |E|$. After compression, the number of nodes is $N_c < N_o$. The *rate of compression*, or *compression ratio*, is $C = 1 - N_c/N_o$.

3.1.1   Lossy Versus Lossless Compression

When a graph $G = (V, E)$ is compressed to form $G' = (V', E')$ and then G' is subsequently decompressed to form $G'' = (V'', E'')$, it is possible that G and G'' are not equal. In particular, it is always true that $V = V''$, however it is possible that $E \neq E''$. If a *lossless* compression method is used then $E = E''$, i.e., the original data is exactly reproduced. In contrast, when *lossy* compression is used then $E \neq E''$ and so G'' is only an approximation of G.

Suppose that nodes n_1 and n_2 in G are merged to form node n, creating the compressed graph G'. Then we have all of the following:

- G' contains all nodes in G, except that nodes n_1 and n_2 in G are replaced by node n in G', i.e., $V' = V - \{n_1, n_2\} \cup \{n\}$.
- All edges of the form (n_1, u) in E, where $u \in V : u \neq n_2$, are replaced by (n, u) in E'.
- All edges of the form (n_2, v) in E, where $v \in V : v \neq n_1$, are replaced by (n, v) in E'.

In the case that n_1 and n_2 both have edges incident with the same other node $u = v$ in G, then when G' is decompressed to form G'' these same edges will appear in G''. In addition, G'' contains the edge (n_1, n_2) because conceptually when n_1 and n_2 are merged they are seen as a clique. Figure 3.1 depicts the situation in which (n_1, n_2), (n_1, u), and (n_2, u) are all edges in the original graph G. In particular, (n_1, n_2), (n_1, n_3), and (n_2, n_3) are all edges in G and neither n_1 nor n_2 have edges to any other node. As a result, G'' still contains this same set of edges. Because $G = G''$, this compression is lossless.

In comparison, when (n_1, u) is in G but (n_2, u) is not, then there will be an additional edge (n_2, u) in G'' that is not in G; similarly, when (n_2, v) is in G but (n_1, v) is not, then there will be an additional edge (n_1, v) in G'' that is not in G. Further, if the edge (n_1, n_2) does not appear in G but n_1 and n_2 are merged, then G'' will contain this additional edge. In these situations, the compression is lossy because $G \neq G''$. The additional edges are called *fake edges* because they appear in G'' but not in the original graph G.

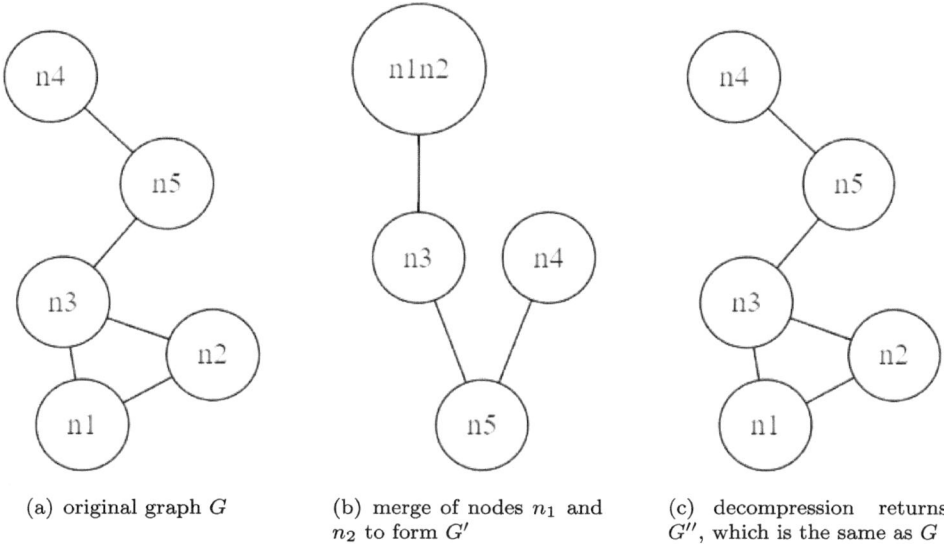

(a) original graph G (b) merge of nodes n_1 and   (c) decompression returns
                                    n_2 to form G' G'', which is the same as G

Fig. 3.1 Compression: merge of two nodes connected by an edge, and with edges to one other common node

Figures 3.2 and 3.3 depict situations in which lossy compression occurs. In Fig. 3.2 nodes n_1 and n_2 are connected by an edge but only n_1 has an edge to node n_3. As a result, when G is compressed by merging n_1 and n_2 then upon subsequent decompression the decompressed graph G'' will contain the fake edge (n_2, n_3) which did not exist in the original graph G. In Fig. 3.3 nodes n_1 and n_2 are not connected by an edge, but both have edges to node n_3. As a result, when G is compressed by merging n_1 and n_2 then upon subsequent decompression the decompressed graph G'' will contain the fake edge (n_1, n_2) which did not exist in the original graph G.

It should be noted that although lossless compression is often considered desirable from the perspective of exactly reproducing the original graph, lossless graph compression algorithms are often very time-consuming. They also may not be able to achieve a high rate of compression. Furthermore, in many cases, it is simply not required that the original graph be exactly reproduced upon decompression. In particular, recall that one of the objectives in using graph compression in epidemic-related research is to compress a very large personal contact network to make it manageable for further analysis. As the objective is to use the compressed graph, an exact reproduction of the original graph is not required. As such, a lossy method that still aims to reduce distortion is a good choice.

It is also important to consider how lossless and lossy compression each handle noise that might appear in data. In the case of a personal contact network, such noise is common. In unweighted graphs, the noise takes the form of missing or extraneous edges or nodes; for weighted graphs, this is extended to also include incorrect edge weights. Since lossless

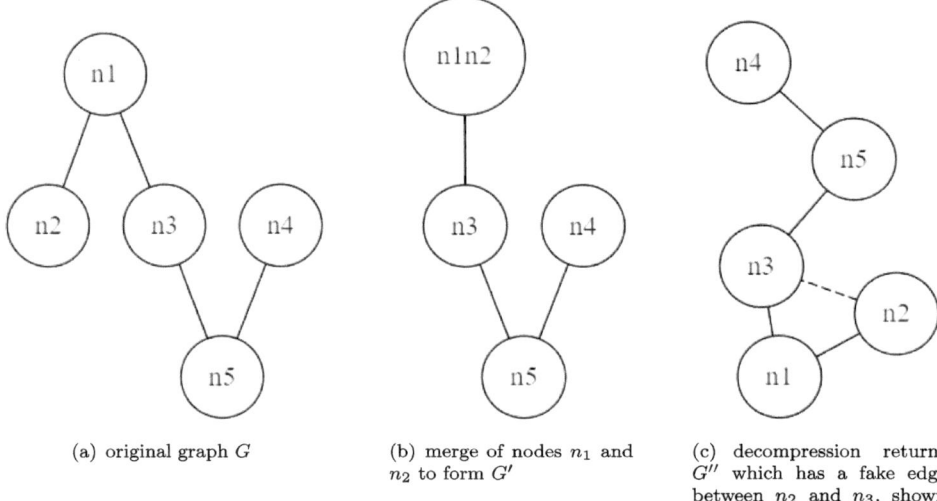

(a) original graph G

(b) merge of nodes n_1 and n_2 to form G'

(c) decompression returns G'' which has a fake edge between n_2 and n_3, shown as a dashed line

Fig. 3.2 Compression: merge of two nodes connected by an edge, with only one having an edge to another node

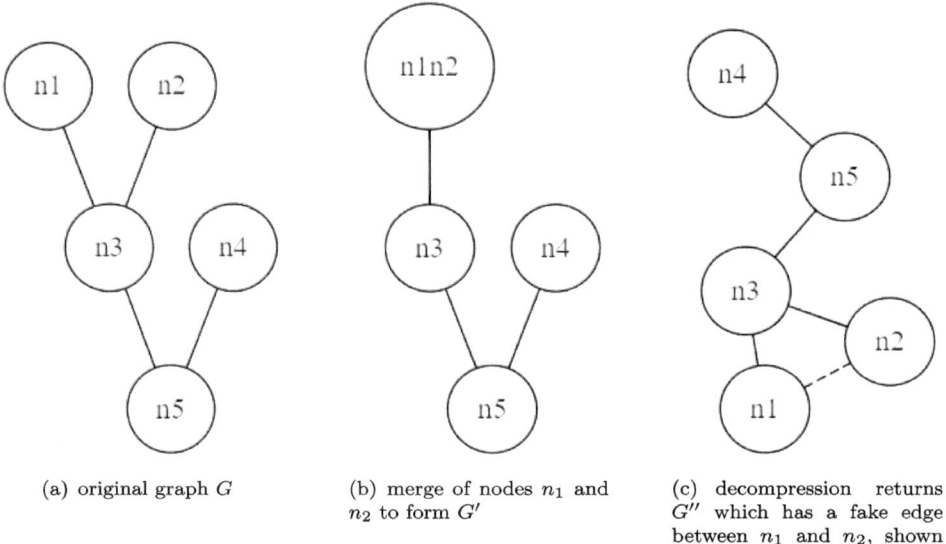

(a) original graph G

(b) merge of nodes n_1 and n_2 to form G'

(c) decompression returns G'' which has a fake edge between n_1 and n_2, shown as a dashed line

Fig. 3.3 Compression: merge of two nodes not connected by an edge, but with edges to one other common node

compression ensures the graph is unaffected by compression and subsequent decompression, any associated noise is maintained. However, lossy compression will tend to ignore noise when seeking strongly-related nodes to merge, as (up to some limit) the noise does not affect the evaluation of which nodes are strongly related.

3.2   Unweighted Graph Compression

The evolutionary algorithm presented here selects pairs of nodes to merge in order to achieve the desired compression ratio, which is provided as input. It is a lossy algorithm, however it still seeks to minimize the amount of distortion created by compression and subsequent decompression. The evolutionary algorithm evolves the choice of which nodes are to be merged according to a fitness function based on minimizing distortion.

3.2.1   Representation

The graph consists of a set of nodes (vertices) V and a set of edges E. Each node can be given a label which is simply an integer in the range $[0, |V| - 1]$. The edges can be stored using an adjacency matrix or adjacency list representation. A graph is considered *dense* if $|E|$ is close to $|V|^2$, i.e., most nodes have edges to most other nodes. A graph is considered *sparse* if $|E| << |V|^2$. Personal contact networks tend to be sparse because most individuals tend to have a small number of contacts relative to the total number of people in the population. For most graph algorithms, the adjacency list representation is preferred for sparse graphs for complexity reasons. It also is preferred for ease of manipulation in the evolutionary algorithm for graph compression.

After compression, each node may be one of the nodes in the original graph, or may be a supernode that is the result of merging two or more of the nodes in the original graph. Suppose that the original graph G has $N_o = |V|$ nodes. For a compression ratio of C, the number of nodes in the graph must be reduced by $l = C \times N_o$ to produce a compressed graph G' with $N_c = N_o - l$ nodes. Each merge combines two nodes into one, thereby reducing the overall number of nodes by one.

The chromosome in the evolutionary algorithm represents the sequence of merges in the compression. As such, the chromosome is of length l. An easy representation is to use a pair of matching arrays, in which the corresponding indices in each of the arrays represents one pair of nodes that are merged.

Index i of the first array, which we call the *root* array, stores the (integer) label of the first node in the ith merge. Index i of the second array records the second node in the ith merge. It must be ensured that the first and second nodes in each merge are always distinct from one another, so that a node is never merged with itself. A simple means of ensuring this is to store the offset of the second node from the first, where each offset is a value in the range $[1, N_o]$. As such, the second array is called the *offset* array. If `root[i]` $= x$ and `offset[i]` $= j$ then nodes x and $y = x + j$ modulo N_o are merged in the ith merge. The label of the supernode created by this merge is set to x. The second node in a merge can be seen as being absorbed into the first node in that merge; although it will be recovered during decompression, it will not be seen directly in the compressed graph.

Figures 3.4 and 3.5 show an example of compression using a compression ratio of 40%. As the initial graph has 10 nodes, a total of 4 merges must occur, thus the chromosome consists of two matching arrays each of length 4. Each of the merges indicated by the chromosome are implemented in turn, with the details of the first 3 merges given in Figs. 3.6, 3.7 and 3.8. Figure 3.6 shows the result of the first merge. According to the chromosome, the root node of this merge has index 3, and the resulting supernode maintains this label. The second node in this merge has index $(3 + 4)\%10 = 7$. Figure 3.7 shows the result of the second merge. As indicated by the chromosome, the root node again has index 3, while the second node has index $(3 + 6)\%10 = 9$. The resulting supernode again has label 3, and because these first two merges build upon each other it is actually the result of merging nodes with indices 3, 7, and 9. Figure 3.8 shows the result of the third merge, in which the root node has index 4 and the other node has index $(4 + 7)\%10 = 1$. The final merge is between nodes with indices 4 (root) and $(4 + 8)\%10 = 2$, and the final result of the entire sequence of merges is shown in Fig. 3.4b.

Each individual merge may contribute to the creation of fake edges once the resulting graph is later decompressed. The result of decompression is shown in Fig. 3.9. For this example, a total of 14 fake edges were created. A lossless compression would result in zero fake edges, although this is rarely feasible. Instead, as will be seen in subsequent sections, one of the goals is to use merges that will minimize the number of fake edges created.

3.2.2   Initial Population

The initial population consists of a set of chromosomes that are randomly generated, subject to the constraints specified above. From the graph point of view, this means that each chromosome in the initial population would represent a sequence of completely random merges in which any node could be merged with any other node in the graph. Although this is easy to implement, it means that nodes may be merged that are far away from each other, in terms of the number of edges traversed to get from one to the other. In the case that we are compressing personal contact networks, the nodes represent individuals, and merging individuals far away from each other makes little sense in terms of personal contact.

A better solution is to require that the nodes in a given merge are within a given distance of each other. This means that the merges are more sensible, in that the nodes are more closely connected. Enforcing this restriction also tends to lead to better fitness, as will be explained in Sect. 3.2.6. For most graphs, a very small distance of no more than 3 would be appropriate, and in fact for personal contact networks distance 1 or 2 works very well

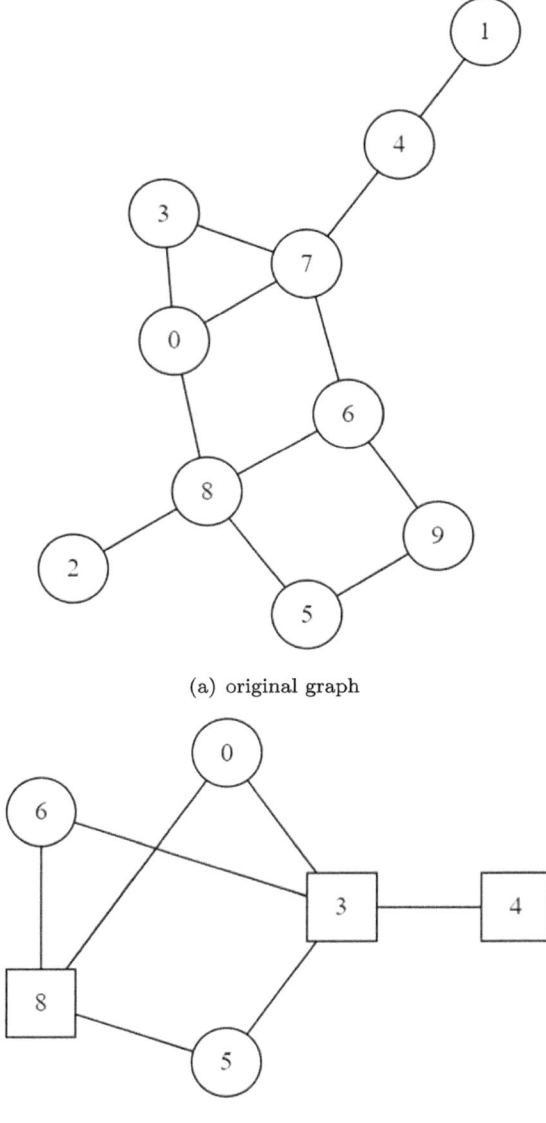

(a) original graph

(b) graph compressed by 40%

Fig. 3.4 Compression of a graph by 40% using the chromosome given in Fig. 3.5. Nodes shown as circles are single unmerged nodes, with the label being the index of that node. Nodes shown as squares are supernodes that are the result of merging two or more nodes, with the label being the index of the root node from the chromosome

(Houghten et al. 2019; Rutkowski et al. 2020). However, this can vary from one type of graph to another, and is an aspect to be carefully considered.

root	3	3	4	8
offset	4	6	7	4

Fig. 3.5 Chromosome used for compression in Fig. 3.4

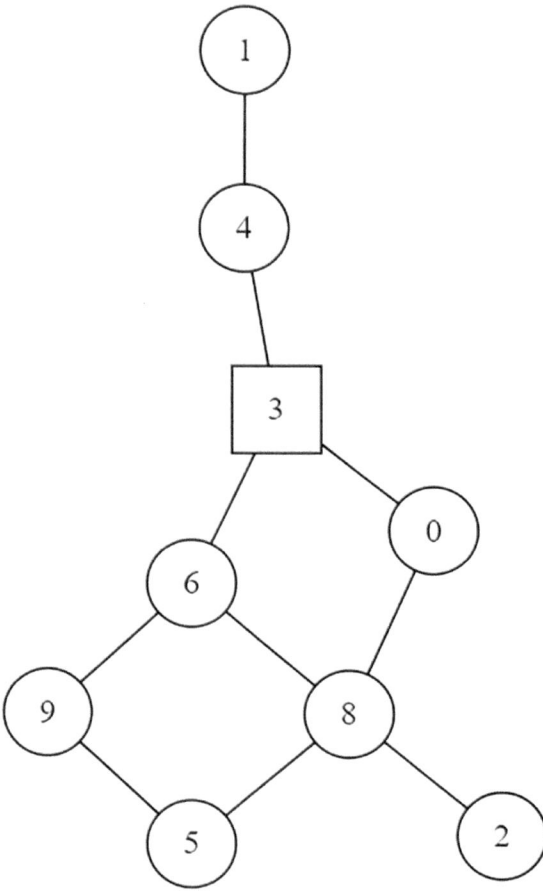

Fig. 3.6 Result of first merge for the initial graph given in Fig. 3.4. Nodes shown as circles are single unmerged nodes, with the label being the index of that node. The node shown as a square is a supernode resulting from merging nodes 3 and 7, and has a label that is the index of the root node (3) for that merge. Note that there is now an edge between node 3 and node 4 because in the original graph there was an edge between node 7 and node 4, and also an edge between node 3 and node 6 because in the original graph there was an edge between node 7 and node 6

To implement this restriction, the initial population is constructed by first randomly generating the entries in the *root* array, i.e., randomly choosing the label of the first node

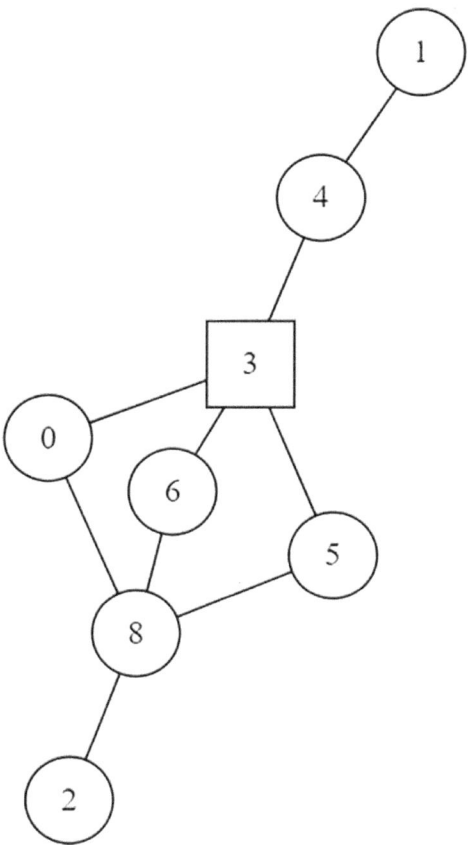

Fig. 3.7 Result of second merge for the initial graph given in Fig. 3.4. This merge occurs upon the graph shown in Fig. 3.6. Nodes shown as circles are single unmerged nodes, with the label being the index of that node. The node shown as a square is the supernode resulting from merging nodes 3 and 9, and has a label that is the index of the root node (3) for that merge. Note that there is now an edge between node 3 and node 5 because in Fig. 3.6 there was an edge between node 9 and node 5

in each of the merges. Given `root[i]` $= x$, a search can be performed from node x to find nodes within the given distance, and then one of these, say y, is randomly chosen to be the node with which x is merged. The value of `offset[i]` is then set to $j = y - x$ modulo N_o. Note that this search can be exhaustive, i.e., a complete breadth-first search to find *all* nodes within the specified distance before making a random choice. Alternatively, some heuristic could be used to examine only certain nodes, thereby greatly speeding up this step; in the extreme, one could simply follow one random path of the appropriate length starting from x to reach (and then choose) y. In examining the example shown in Figs. 3.4, 3.5, 3.6, 3.7, 3.8 and 3.9, the second merge would not be allowed if the distance restriction were set to one.

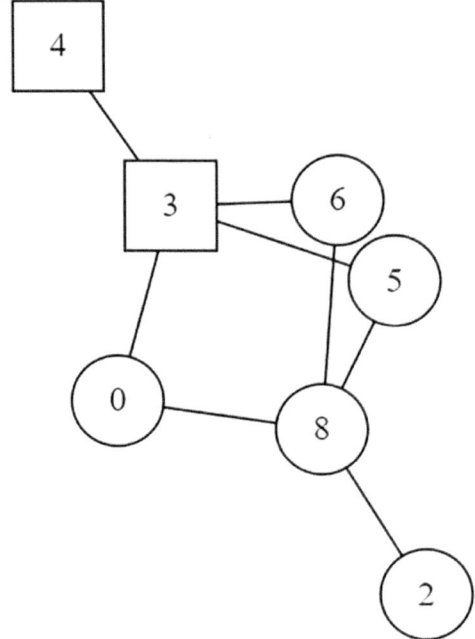

Fig. 3.8 Result of third merge for the initial graph given in Fig. 3.4. This merge occurs upon the graph shown in Fig. 3.7. Nodes shown as circles are single unmerged nodes, with the label being the index of that node. The node shown as a square with label 4 is the supernode resulting from merging nodes 4 and 1, and has the label 4 because it is the index of the root node for that merge

3.2.3 Selection

To select the two parents for reproduction, tournament selection can be used. If this is used, then a separate tournament selection process should take place for each parent. For this process, k chromosomes should be randomly chosen from the population and evaluated based on their fitness. The best of these chromosomes is then selected as one of the parents, and the process is repeated for the second parent.

Crossover and mutation are then applied to these parents, as described in the following subsections, to create two child chromosomes. The overall process is repeated multiple times to create all chromosomes for the next generation.

3.2.4 Crossover

Crossover creates two children by randomly choosing one or more points within the chromosome. The first child receives a copy of all entries from the first parent up to the first crossover point, all entries from the second parent from the first crossover point to the second, and continuing to alternate in this fashion until the end of the chromosome. The second child receives a copy of all entries from the parents that are not in the first child.

Recall that the size of the chromosome is $N_o - N_c$. If two-point crossover is used then the first crossover point is a random value between 1 and $N_o - N_c$, and the second crossover point is a random value between the first crossover point and $N_o - N_c$. If using the representation described in Sect. 3.2.1 then crossover is applied simultaneously to both arrays.

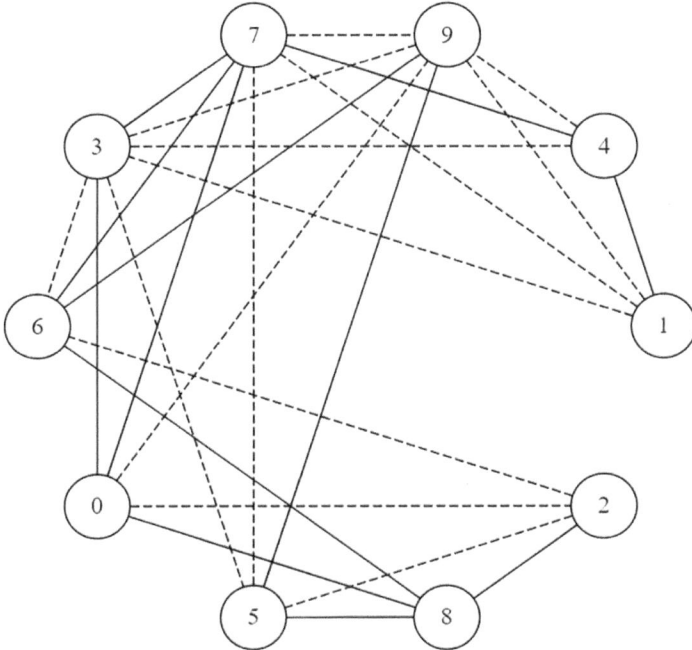

Fig. 3.9 Graph resulting from decompression of the final graph given in Fig. 3.4. Fake edges are shown as dashed lines

3.2.5   Mutation

Mutation randomly changes some of the information contained in the chromosome. For this application, single-point mutation is an appropriate choice. In single-point mutation, a location is randomly chosen in the chromosome and the value at that location is modified.

The effect of mutation is to change a single merge. Assuming the representation described in Sect. 3.2.1, mutation must be applied simultaneously to both arrays. The mutation point is chosen randomly as a value j between 1 and $N_o - N_c$, and `root[j]` is set to a random value between 0 and $N_o - 1$, which changes the first node in the jth merge. The entry in `offset[j]` can similarly be set to a random value between 1 and N_o, thereby randomly changing the second node in the jth merge. However, if we want to ensure that only nodes within a given distance are merged then we need to follow the same process described in Sect. 3.2.2 to choose a second node that is within that distance.

3.2.6 Fitness Function

In compressing the graph, the overall size is reduced but as noted in Sect. 3.1.1, some distortion may be introduced. Since the methodology takes the desired compression ratio as input, the fitness is based on minimizing the amount of distortion introduced during the process.[1] To minimize distortion, the fitness function is based on merging nodes with a high level of "similarity", although similarity may be defined in different ways. Each individual merge contributes to the overall fitness.

Consider the merging of two nodes n_1 and n_2. In general, we would want to reward merges of nodes that have a high number of adjacent nodes in common, as such nodes can be seen as similar to one another. Another consideration is to reward merges of nodes that are neighbours of one another, because such nodes can be seen to be closely related. A fitness function taking these two considerations into account was presented in Brown et al. (2016). If L_1 is the set of nodes adjacent to n_1 and L_2 is the set of nodes adjacent to n_2 then the fitness associated with the merge of n_1 and n_2 is $|L_1 \cap L_2| + bonus$, where $bonus$ is a value designed to reward merges of nodes that are neighbours: $bonus = 0$ if n_1 and n_2 are not neighbours, and is a positive constant value otherwise.

In this chapter we use a more general fitness function that uses the concept of *fake edges* described in Sect. 3.1.1. In so doing, this fitness function actually tends to reward merges of nodes that have many adjacent nodes in common. In addition, if the selection and mutation processes merge nodes within a given (small) distance of each other then such merges would also often be rewarded with the *bonus* specified above. As fake edges do not appear in the original graph, but do appear in the graph that results from compression followed by decompression, they are a form of distortion that should be minimized. As such, the fitness function is a simple count of the number of fake edges created by the sequence of merges, and a lower fitness value is better.

Consider again the example chromosome shown in Fig. 3.5. Using this chromosome, the initial graph G shown in the top of Fig. 3.4 is compressed to produce the compressed graph G' shown in the bottom of Fig. 3.4. Decompression then produces the graph G'' shown in Fig. 3.9, which has a total of 13 fake edges, i.e., the fitness of this solution is 13.

---

[1] An alternative would be to decide upon an acceptable amount of distortion, and work towards maximizing the compression possible for that distortion. Fitness would then be based on maximizing the compression ratio. This is a more complicated alternative, however, since the chromosomes would vary in length.

3.2.7 Multi-objective Algorithm

The single-objective algorithm shown above requires a target compression ratio, which determines the number of merges to be performed. The algorithm then works to find sequences of merges that minimize the amount of distortion created during the compression. This is sensible if the user already has a desired target compression in mind, but this target is not always clear. For example, a user may simply say that they want the compressed graph to be "as small as possible"—at the extreme, this would mean that all nodes in the graph would be merged to form a single supernode, with an accompanying extremely high level of distortion. At the other extreme, the user may request zero distortion, which in general is only possible for a very small compression ratio. For most graphs and applications, neither option is desirable. A multi-objective algorithm allows us to see the trade-off between compression ratio and distortion.

A multi-objective algorithm based on NSGA-II (Deb et al. 2002) was applied to the problem of compression of large networks in Collins et al. (2017). In this, it was demonstrated that the multi-objective algorithm could be used to select an appropriate target compression ratio. Once this was selected, the single objective algorithm could be applied to this target. Following this process led to significantly better results than simply using the multi-objective algorithm for the given compression ratio. Effectively, the single-objective GA was able to focus all of its efforts on the given target, while the multi-objective GA spread its efforts, examining multiple targets.

3.3 Weighted Graph Compression

Sometimes we would like a personal contact network to represent not only which individuals in a population are in contact with one another, but also the strength of their connection. To do so, a *weighted* graph is used. As described in Sect. 3.2.1 for unweighted graphs, either an adjacency list or adjacency matrix representation can also be used for weighted graphs.

A weighted personal contact network is a weighted graph in which the weight of edge (u, v) indicates the level of contact between individuals u and v. If the weight is zero then this indicates that u and v do not have any contact with each other, while a higher positive weight indicates a stronger connection. Note that in this context, no weights can be negative. The values of the weights can be determined in multiple ways. A simple representation might simply allocate values according to a set of predefined classes: for example: {0 = no contact, 1 = rare contact, 2 = workplace or school contact, 3 = household contact}. Some studies (Isella 2011; SocioPatterns 2009, 2021) have used sensors that detect when individuals come into contact, as measured by being within a given distance of each other. Using such data, the weight could be a simple count of, or some calculation based upon, the number of times the individuals come into contact during a given time frame (Rutkowski et al. 2020).

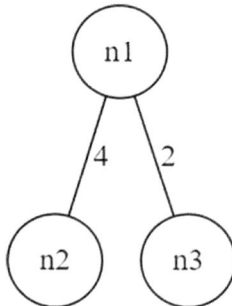

Fig. 3.10 Example of a weighted graph

Regardless of the method used to assign weights, it is important for the end user to decide on the appropriate level of granularity for their application.

Consider the example shown in Fig. 3.10. If this graph were obtained by a count of the number of times each pair of individuals were in contact during a given time period, then this graph indicates that the individuals represented by nodes n_1 and n_2 were in contact four times, n_1 and n_3 were in contact two times, and n_2 and n_3 had no contact. If n_1 were infected, then there would be four opportunities for them to pass infection to n_2 and two opportunities for them to pass it to n_3. In contrast, if n_2 were infected then they could not pass the infection directly to n_3, but it could pass from n_2 to n_1 and then onwards to n_3. We will use this graph to display the outcomes of compression in the following sections.

3.3.1   Changes in Edge Weights During Compression and Decompression

The method presented for compression of unweighted graphs has a fitness function based on changes in the connectivity of the graph, i.e., additional (*fake*) edges created, when the graph is compressed and then subsequently decompressed. When compressing and then decompressing a weighted graph, the process may also introduce another form of distortion, namely changes in edge weights.

Before considering a possible fitness function, we first need to consider how the edges and their weights are affected during compression and decompression. A detailed study on this topic is presented in Toivonen (2011). Consider the three examples shown in Figs. 3.11, 3.12, and 3.13, that demonstrate the results of the three different options for a single merge on the same initial graph G.

In Fig. 3.11, in the original graph G nodes n_1 and n_2 are connected by an edge of weight 4, and nodes n_1 and n_3 are connected by an edge of weight 2. When G is compressed by merging n_1 and n_2 then the resulting supernode n_1n_2 in the compressed graph G' has an "internal edge" of weight 4. This represents the fact that the nodes which form the supernode (in this case n_1 and n_2) are a clique in which every edge has weight 4. The compressed graph

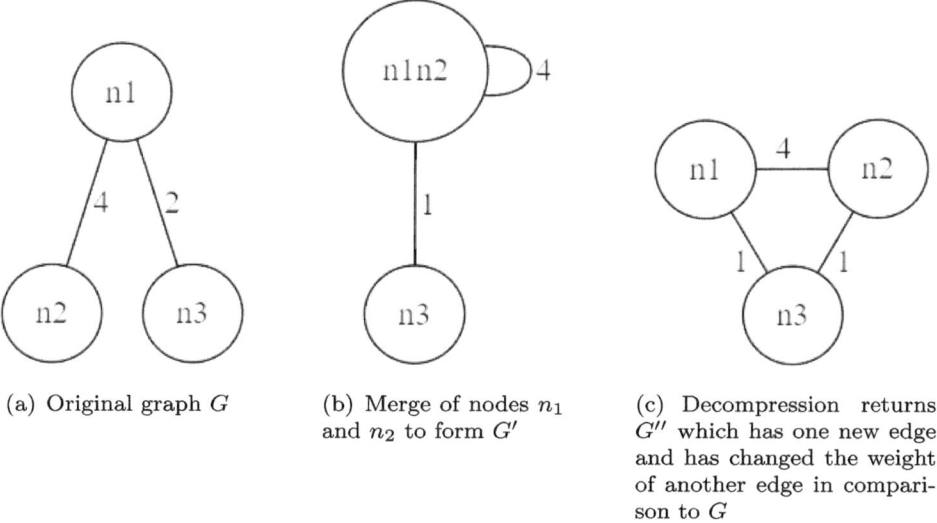

(a) Original graph G

(b) Merge of nodes n_1 and n_2 to form G'

(c) Decompression returns G'' which has one new edge and has changed the weight of another edge in comparison to G

Fig. 3.11 Compression of a weighted graph: first option

G' also has an edge between $n_1 n_2$ and n_3 of weight 1—this is the average weight, in the original graph G, of edge (n_1, n_3) (namely, 2) and edge (n_2, n_3) (namely, 0, since this edge did not exist in G). When G' is subsequently decompressed to form G'', edge (n_1, n_2) has weight 4, obtained from the internal weight of the supernode in the compressed graph G', and the edges (n_1, n_3) and (n_2, n_3) both have weight 1, obtained from the weight of the edge $(n_1 n_2, n_3)$ in the compressed graph G'.

In Fig. 3.12, when G is compressed by merging nodes n_1 and n_3 then the resulting supernode $n_1 n_3$ in the compressed graph G' has an "internal edge" with weight 2. The edge $(n_1 n_3, n_2)$ has weight 2 because this is the average weight, in the original graph G, of edge (n_1, n_2) (namely, 4) and edge (n_2, n_3) (namely, 0 since it did not exist in G). When G' is subsequently decompressed to form G'', edge (n_1, n_3) has weight 2, obtained from the internal weight of the supernode in the compressed graph G', and the edges (n_1, n_2) and (n_2, n_3) both have weight 2, obtained from the weight of the edge $(n_1 n_3, n_2)$ in the compressed graph G'.

Figure 3.13 depicts a situation in which the merged nodes were not originally directly connected by an edge. In this example, when G is compressed by merging nodes n_2 and n_3 then the resulting supernode $n_2 n_3$ in the compressed graph G' has an "internal edge" with weight 0, which in our application represents a non-existent edge.[2] The edge $(n_2 n_3, n_1)$ has weight 3 because this is the average weight, in the original graph G, of edges (n_1, n_2) (namely, 4) and (n_1, n_3) (namely, 2). When G' is subsequently decompressed to form G'',

---

[2] In a personal contact network, it is appropriate for an edge of weight zero to denote that there is zero contact between those two individuals. It is important to recognize that in other applications, there may be weights that have a negative or zero value and the meaning of the edge weights may be different. Such applications could require changes to the process.

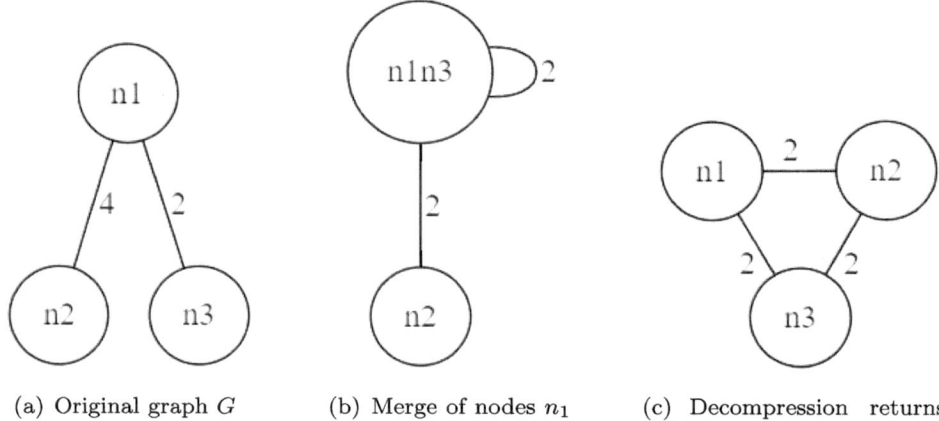

(a) Original graph G

(b) Merge of nodes n_1 and n_2 to form G'

(c) Decompression returns G'' which has one new edge and has changed the weight of another edge in comparison to G

Fig. 3.12 Compression of a weighted graph: second option

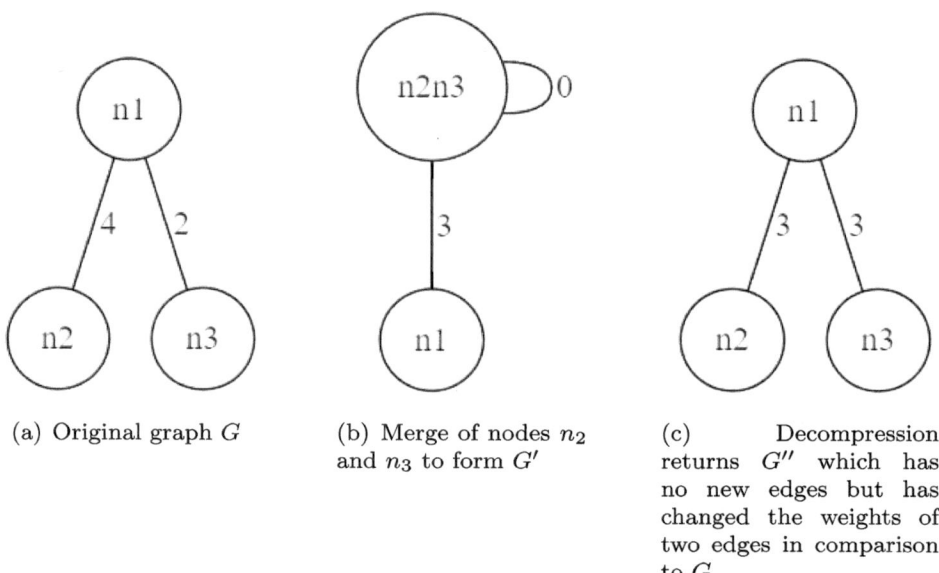

(a) Original graph G

(b) Merge of nodes n_2 and n_3 to form G'

(c) Decompression returns G'' which has no new edges but has changed the weights of two edges in comparison to G

Fig. 3.13 Compression of a weighted graph: third option

edges (n_1, n_2) and (n_1, n_3) both have weight 3, obtained from the weight of the edge $(n_2n_3, n_1$ in the compressed graph G'. Also, because the supernode (n_2n_3) in the compressed graph G' has weight 0, when decompressed this means there is no edge (or equivalently for this application, an edge of weight 0) between nodes n_2 and n_3.

3.3.2 Fitness Function

The fitness function must be modified to account for changes in both the structure and the edge weights of the graph when graph G is compressed and then subsequently decompressed to produce G''. In fact since we are using an edge weight of zero to indicate the nonexistence of an edge, if a new ("fake") edge is created from node u to node v then this will show up as a change in edge weight for the edge (u, v) from zero to a positive value. As such, the fitness function can simply use changes in edge weight to evaluate both kinds of changes in the graph. As for the unweighted graphs, the evolutionary algorithm should aim to minimize the value returned by the fitness function.

The first fitness function, presented in Rutkowski et al. (2020) is based upon the total absolute difference between the weights in G and G'', considering every pair of nodes u and v. This function is calculated as $fitness = \sum_{u,v \in G} |wt(u, v) - wt''(u, v)|$, where $wt(u, v)$ denotes the weight of the edge (u, v) in G and $wt''(u, v)$ denotes the weight of the edge (u, v) in G''. Recall that if there is no edge between u and v then it is treated as an edge that has weight zero.

Consider the examples shown in Figs. 3.11, 3.12, and 3.13. For each of these, the fitness is $|wt(n_1, n_2) - wt''(n_1, n_2)| + |wt(n_1, n_3) - wt''(n_1, n_3)| + |wt(n_2, n_3) - wt''(n_2, n_3)|$. The compression shown in Fig. 3.11, in which the merge was between two nodes connected by a high-weight edge, has a fitness of 2. In contrast, the compression shown in Fig. 3.12, in which the merge was between two nodes connected by a lower-weight edge, has a fitness of 4. The compression shown in Fig. 3.13, which merges two nodes which both share an edge to a common third node, does not create any additional edges and also has a fitness of 2. Thus although each of these examples introduced two modifications during the process of compression and decompression, the middle example is considered a worse compression in terms of this fitness function.

A second possible fitness function, based upon the work presented in Toivonen (2011), is similar to Euclidean distance. This function is calculated as $fitness = \sqrt{\sum_{u,v \in G} (wt(u, v) - wt''(u, v))^2}$, using the same notation as above.

Again consider the examples shown in Figs. 3.11, 3.12, and 3.13. For each of these, the fitness is calculated as

$$\sqrt{(wt(n_1, n_2) - wt''(n_1, n_2))^2 + (wt(n_1, n_3) - wt''(n_1, n_3))^2 + (wt(n_2, n_3) - wt''(n_2, n_3))^2}.$$

Again the compressions shown in Figs. 3.11 and 3.13 both have the best fitness, in this case $\sqrt{2}$, while the compression given in Fig. 3.12 has a fitness of $\sqrt{8}$.

With respect to a personal contact network, this implies that merging two nodes that represent two strongly-connected individuals, or merging two nodes that have another contact in common, would both be preferred over merging two nodes that represent two weakly-connected individuals. In terms of the goal stated at the start of this chapter of simplifying the personal contact network to produce a "big picture" view for further analysis, a compression that favours such choices makes sense. A comparison of these two fitness functions, along with a comparison to the Louvain algorithm for community detection in weighted graphs, is performed on weighted contact network data in Rutkowski et al. (2021). The results showed that using weighted edges significantly added detail and affected the actual merges used in the compression.

All other aspects of the evolutionary algorithm presented in Sect. 3.2 for unweighted graph compression can be used for weighted graph compression. Although it is not presented here, it is also possible to develop a multi-objective algorithm for compression of weighted graphs, as for unweighted graphs.

References

J.A. Brown, S. Houghtent, T.K. Collins, Q. Qu, Evolving graph compression using similarity measures for bioinformatics applications, in *2016 IEEE Conference on Computational Intelligence in Bioinformatics and Computational Biology (CIBCB)* (2016), pp. 1–6. https://doi.org/10.1109/CIBCB.2016.7758126

T.K. Collins, A. Zakirov, J.A. Brown, S. Houghten, Single-objective and multi-objective genetic algorithms for compression of biological networks, in *2017 IEEE Conference on Computational Intelligence in Bioinformatics and Computational Biology (CIBCB)* (2017), pp. 1–8. https://doi.org/10.1109/CIBCB.2017.8058564

K. Deb, A. Pratap, S. Agarwal, T. Meyarivan, A fast and elitist multiobjective genetic algorithm: Nsga-ii. IEEE Trans. Evolu. Comput. **6**(2), 182–197 (2002). ISSN 1089-778X. https://doi.org/10.1109/4235.996017

S. Houghten, A. Romualdo, T.K. Collins, J.A. Brown, Compression of biological networks using a genetic algorithm with localized merge, in *2019 IEEE Conference on Computational Intelligence in Bioinformatics and Computational Biology (CIBCB)* (2019), pp. 1–8. https://doi.org/10.1109/CIBCB.2019.8791490

L. Isella et al., What's in a crowd? Analysis of face-to-face behavioral networks. J. Theor. Biol. **271**(1), 166–180 (2011). ISSN 0022-5193 https://doi.org/10.1016/j.jtbi.2010.11.033. http://www.sciencedirect.com/science/article/B6WMD-51M60KS-2/2/cb31bee32b340b3044c724b88779a60e

E. Rutkowski, S. Houghten, J.A. Brown, Extracting information from weighted contact networks via genetic algorithms, in *2020 IEEE Conference on Computational Intelligence in Bioinformatics and Computational Biology (CIBCB)* (2020), pp. 1–8. https://doi.org/10.1109/CIBCB48159.2020.9277709

E. Rutkowski, J. Sargant, S. Houghten, J.A. Brown, Evaluation of communities from exploratory evolutionary compression of weighted graphs, in *2021 IEEE Congress on Evolutionary Computation (CEC)* (2021), pp. 434–441. https://doi.org/10.1109/CEC45853.2021.9504833

SocioPatterns. Deployment: Infectious SocioPatterns (2009). http://www.sociopatterns.org/deployments/infectious-sociopatterns/

SocioPatterns. Infectious contact networks (2021). http://www.sociopatterns.org/datasets/

H. Toivonen et al., Compression of weighted graphs, in *Proceedings of the 17th ACM SIGKDD International Conference on Knowledge Discovery and Data Mining* (2011), pp. 965–973

Ideally, contact tracing would be done for all virus cases and we would be able to use the results to build a network on which different mediation strategies could be simulated. Unfortunately, for the COVID-19 pandemic (and many other infectious diseases), this did not happen. Some contact tracing was done, both electronically and using the *old-fashioned in-person method*, but privacy concerns prevented even this from being available to researchers. So, in order to develop and test our mediation strategies, we need plausible contact networks. We create these from the case data using an evolutionary algorithm.

4.1   Evolutionary Algorithm

Darwin, who discovered the idea of natural selection, offers us the foundation for the ideas used in evolutionary computation (Darwin 1909). He observed that random minor alterations to a species, across time, permitted some members of the population to outlive others, and eventually causing more members of the species to acquire said alteration. Those who had the modification would have more offspring, live longer, and/or be more fit for the environment which granted those genes a greater chance of reproductive success. Across successive generations of the species those without the modification would die off, while those with the modification would thrive. This process is constantly occurring in all biological systems and is the basis for the diversity that exists in nature. The successive advances in living organisms are indirectly stored in the DNA that codes the cells and proteins that comprise the organisms (Futuyma and Kirkpatrick 2017).

In order to simulate this evolution a problem and its potential solutions (known as *chromosomes*) must be stored in the computer in a manner which allows for evolution. This includes how candidate solutions are *represented*, *initialized*, *selected* for reproduction,

J. Hughes et al., *AI Versus Epidemics*, Synthesis Lectures on Learning,
Networks, and Algorithms, https://doi.org/10.1007/978-3-031-64373-6_4

undergo *reproduction*, experience *mutation*, and are *evaluated* in comparison to one another (Russell and Norvig 2016). An evolutionary algorithm will be used to generate plausible personal contact networks which can be used to simulate epidemics likely to result in particular outcomes, dependant on the chosen evaluation metric.

4.1.1 Representation

The first hurdle to using evolutionary algorithms on a test problem is choosing a suitable representation for potential solutions (the chromosomes) to the problem. Like DNA in living things, this representation must be robust enough to represent any and all potential solutions to the problem at hand. Typically, a string of letters and/or numbers are used to represent a solution within the algorithm with rules to convert the string representation to a solution to the real-world problem being solved (Russell and Norvig 2016). In this case, a representation capable of specifying a personal contact network is required.

Our evolutionary algorithm evolves lists of edge operations that will be applied to an initial network. Each edge operation either adds, deletes, or moves edges within the network. Applying each edge operation to the initial network sequentially results in a unique final network. Thus, the algorithm is searching for the best list of edge operations to apply to the initial network. The best list creates a final network which, when evaluated, has the best fitness value. Next, a variety of initial networks will be outlined before the edge operations are introduced.

4.1.1.1 Initial Network

Our algorithm determines the best edge modifications to be made to the provided initial network. The initial network has an impact on the properties of the final network. This is partly a result of the exponential variety of potential networks which can exists, especially as the number of nodes, N, within the network increases. If an undirected network has N nodes then there are a total of $N(N-1)/2$ potential edges within the network as each node could be connected to each of the other $N-1$ nodes. This results in a total of $2^{(N(N-1)/2)}$ potential networks, as each edge has two choices: it can either exist or not exist in the network. For example, if there are $N = 10$ nodes in a network there are $10(10-1)/2 = 45$ potential edges in the network resulting in $2^{45} = 35, 184, 372, 088, 832$ potential networks. Of course, many of these networks would be uninteresting and/or not useful, i.e. networks with fewer edges than nodes, networks with nodes that have no edges, networks that are *disconnected*, etc. Disconnected networks are graphs where a path of edges does not exist between every pair of nodes in the network. Even with these networks excluded the number of potential networks remains incredibly large. Therefore, the choice of initial network is important because it helps to ensure that the networks generated by the algorithm are representative of the true social networks which exist in human populations. Most public health research collects the number of social contacts each individual within the population has, rather than the specific topology of the network, in terms of which individuals are in direct contact with others. Specifically, research into the number of sexual contacts between individuals shows that there are a few members of the population with hundreds of contacts while the rest of the population has significantly fewer contacts down to one or two for some individuals (Latora et al. 2006; Liljeros et al. 2001). Therefore, it is helpful to start with a network that is 'close' to the actual personal contact networks that exists for a population. This allows us to make a reasonable choice of starting network, namely one where the average degree of the nodes is four or five and a limited number of nodes have a degree much larger than this average.

The first network that has been extensively used in our body of work is known as the *ring network*, seen in Fig. 4.1. Each node in this network has a total of four edges: one to each of the two nodes preceding it and one to each of the two nodes proceeding it. Though this type of structure is unlikely to occur in real personal contact networks, it provided a good baseline to develop the system. The majority of our work uses this as one of the initial networks tested as it allows for a consistent baseline to judge the system's performance.

The other initial networks that have been used to test our system are defined by the methods used to generate them, rather than a set structure like seen in the ring network. These methods are stochastic, meaning the networks they generate are random, though the methods dictate some properties of resultant network. The first such network is known as a *PowerLaw cluster graph*, which is created by adding nodes to an initially empty network one-by-one (Albert and Barabasi 2002). The method used to generate these networks has three parameters: the number of nodes to add to the network, a number of edges to add for each node added to the network, ea, and the probability, p, of adding an extra edge to form a triangle for each edge added according to the previous parameter. The method works by adding a node to the network, n_i, and then connecting this node to ea randomly selected nodes already in the network. This is done by selecting a random node, n_j such that $0 <= j < i$, and adding the edge n_i, n_j if it is not already present in the network. If

Fig. 4.1 Initial graph with 128 vertices on which to apply the string of edge operations. Each vertex has two edges to the two preceding nodes as well as two edges to the two proceeding nodes in the ring

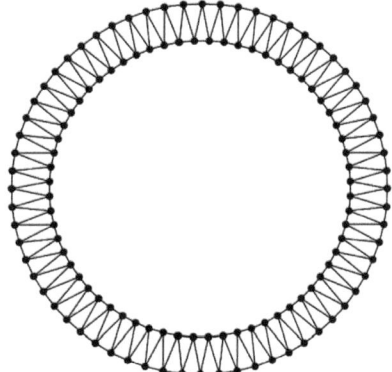

Fig. 4.2 The initial powerlaw
cluster graph with 160 nodes
that strings of edge-editing
operations are applied to

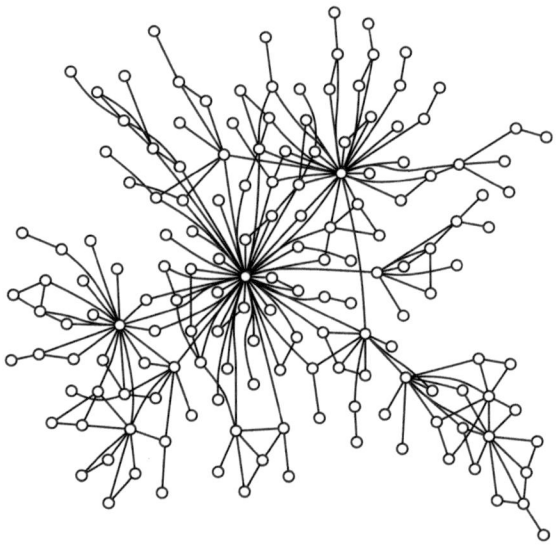

there are sufficient nodes already in the network, $i > ea$, then ea edges are guaranteed to
be added to the network. For each edge added in this manner, there is probability p that a
second edge will be added between node n_j and a node adjacent to n_i, denoted n_k; thus the
additional edge would be edge n_j, n_k. Should this occur, then a *triangle* would be formed
within the network. A triangle is when a triple of nodes exists where each of the three nodes
has an edge from it to the other two nodes in the triple.

This method results in networks that have a few nodes with a large degree, typically 10–
20 times the average degree of the network, while the rest of the nodes are adjacent to only
a handful of nodes. This models the patterns seen in networks of sexual contacts discussed
above. For it's similarity to patterns seen in real life, the PowerLaw cluster graph is a decent
choice of initial network. An example of a PowerLaw cluster graph used in our work is
shown in Fig. 4.2. This graph was generated using the parameters: 160 nodes, $ea = 1$ edge
added for each added node, and triangle probability of $p = 50\%$.

4.1.1.2 Local THADS-N Representation
Once the initial network has been determined the edge-editing commands and how they are
applied will be outlined. This is titled the Local THADS-N representation and it is used to
generate personal contact networks using an initial network, provided as a system parameter,
which will be subject to a list of editing commands to generate a resultant network. These
resultant networks are the output of the system. Thus, the chromosomes that are being
evolved are the lists of edge operations to be applied to the initial network sequentially.
These lists are comprised of some number of *edge-editing operations*, selected from the list
of nine edge-editing operations found in Fig. 4.3. In essence, the system is attempting to

- **Toggle**(p, q): If edge $\{p, q\}$ is in E then remove $\{p, q\}$ from E, otherwise add $\{p, q\}$ to E.

- **Local Toggle**(p, q, r): If edge $\{p, q\}$ and $\{q, r\}$ are in E then **Toggle**(p, r).

- **Hop**(p, q, r): If edge $\{p, q\}$ and $\{q, r\}$ are in E and edge $\{p, r\}$ is not in E then remove edge $\{p, q\}$ from E and add edge $\{p, r\}$ to E.

- **Add**(p, q): If $\{p, q\}$ is not in E then add $\{p, q\}$ to E, otherwise do nothing.

- **Local Add**(p, q, r): If edge $\{p, q\}$ and $\{q, r\}$ are in E then **Add**(p, r).

- **Delete**(p, q): If $\{p, q\}$ is in E then remove $\{p, q\}$ from E, otherwise do nothing.

- **Local Delete**(p, q, r): If edge $\{p, q\}$ and $\{q, r\}$ are in E then **Delete**(p, r).

- **Swap**(p, q, r, s): If $\{p, q\}$ and $\{r, s\}$ are the only edges between p, q, r and s then remove $\{p, q\}$ and $\{r, s\}$ from E and add $\{p, s\}$ and $\{q, r\}$ to E.

- **Null**(): Do nothing.

Fig. 4.3 Given a graph $G(V, E)$ and the vertices p, q, r, and s from the set V the edge-editing operations are defined below

find the optimal list of edge operations to apply to the initial network, so that the resultant network performs the best according to the fitness metric being used, see Sect. 4.1.3. Our work used lists of length 256, though this is a tuneable parameters; in general the number of operations should be twice the number of nodes in the initial network. This is because the number of edge operations in a chromosome determines the achievable difference between the initial and resultant networks. A lower achievable difference means less ability to search the space of all potential solutions; structurally limiting the usefulness of the evolutionary algorithm. The issue of exploring the solution space (all the possible networks with the provided number of nodes) is explored in Chap. 6.

4.1.2 Initialization

The system must determine how to generate the initial population of chromosomes which are evolved during evolution. Initializing an evolutionary algorithm with solutions close to the optimal solution, should one exist, dramatically reduces the time to find said solution as the final population of chromosomes remains close to the initial population. However, the ability to do so depends heavily on the problem being solved and the representation being used. Our system randomly generates the initial population of 1000 solutions according to a probability distribution, provided as a parameter. This distribution determines the likelihood of selecting each of the edge-editing operations during initialization (Table 4.1).

Table 4.1 Example probability distributions for edge-editing operations from Vega Jimenez et al. (2021)

Togg.	Hop	Add	Del.	Swap	L-Togg.	L-Add	L-Del.	Null
0.0438	0.0188	0.0281	0.0499	0.0003	0.4322	0.0051	0.017	0.4047
0.0038	0.0156	0.0221	0.0021	0.0285	0.0267	0.4183	0.0396	0.4432
0.0341	0.0192	0.0044	0.2095	0.0586	0.3328	0.3232	0.0047	0.0134
0.0176	0.3765	0.0125	0.0157	0.3637	0.0094	0.1757	0.0099	0.019
0.3572	0.2016	0.0045	0.0079	0.0026	0.0088	0.3556	0.051	0.0109
0.0122	0.0196	0.3838	0.0942	0.0069	0.0067	0.0303	0.0173	0.4288
0.0038	0.0457	0.4066	0.0769	0.0226	0.0061	0.3952	0.0268	0.0164
0.002	0.0727	0.001	0.0435	0.0355	0.0123	0.7945	0.0201	0.0184

4.1.3   Fitness Evaluation

In order to evaluate the networks generated by the evolutionary algorithm a fitness metric is required. The metric must provide a numerical value representing the relative usefulness of a potential solution. This allows the algorithm to rank the solutions and therefore, determine which of the networks are preferable to reproduce. This metric is what facilitates the gradual improvement of solutions throughout evolution. Our work has used a variety of fitness functions, including: *epidemic length*, *profile matching*, and *epidemic spread*. All of these functions work by simulating multiple epidemics on a potential solution. This is done because an epidemic is stochastic in nature; coming in contact with an infected individual does not guarantee the disease spreads. Several variables impact the chance of this spread, such as length of the interaction, the physical space of the interaction, and your immune system. In order to address the variability of any one epidemic, several independent epidemics are simulated on the networks with their statistics being averaged to determine the value returned by the fitness function. The epidemic length and spread fitness functions simulate between 1 and 5 epidemics, determined by the programmer, whereas profile matching simulates 50 epidemics. The reason for this difference is explained below.

A single simulated epidemic starts by marking all the nodes in the network as susceptible. Then one node, *patient zero*, is selected to be marked infected. In our work, this has been the node with index zero. Each time step, every node adjacent to at least one infected node has a chance of becoming infected by each of their infected neighbours. The likelihood of this infection spreading along each edge connecting a susceptible individual to an infected one is a system parameter α which has typically been set to 0.50. Each such edge is calculated independently, leading to an increased likelihood of infection with the number of adjacent infected nodes. After new infections have been determined, those who are currently infected are marked recovered concluding the current time step. This process continues until there are no remaining infected individuals in the network, indicating end of the epidemic.

The first fitness function, epidemic duration fitness, returns the mean length of the simulated epidemics. The length of a single epidemic is the number of time steps between infecting patient zero and there being no remaining infected individuals. Next, the profile matching fitness function compares the number of infected individuals for each time step to that of a provided epidemic profile. The profiles used in our work are available in Fig. 4.4. The value returned is the average root mean square error between the epidemic curves and the profile being matched. Finally, the epidemic spread fitness function is the average number of infections which occur during the simulated epidemics. The duration and spread functions are to be maximized during evolution whereas the profile matching function is to be minimized.

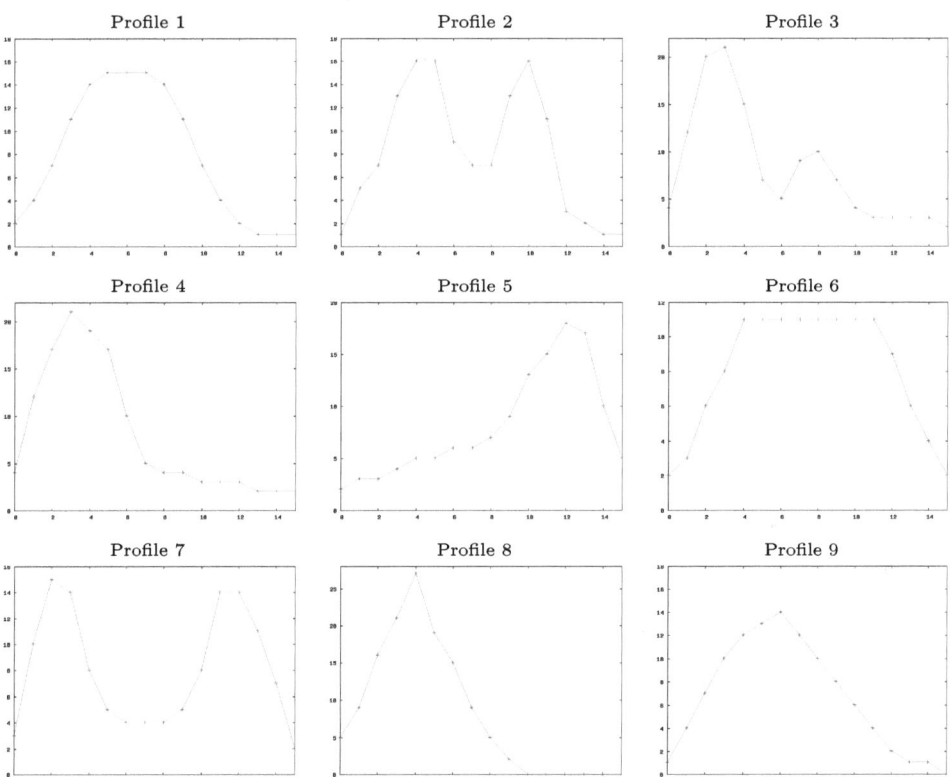

Fig. 4.4 Epidemic profiles representing time step versus number of infected individuals during that time step

4.1.4 Selection

The evolutionary algorithm performs some number of mating events, depending on the fitness function being used. Epidemic duration and spread has typically required 500 000 mating events, while profile matching needed far less at 40 000 mating events. These were sufficient as the improvement in the fitness of the solutions diminishes beyond this number of mating events. The reason for the 10-fold difference in the number of mating events between he fitness functions will be explained below. Each mating event first *selects* certain members of the population to undergo reproduction, then generates new solutions via reproduction, and randomly mutates these new solutions. Profile matching fitness has successfully used size-seven tournament selection in which seven solutions are randomly selected and sorted according to their fitness. The two networks with best fitness are selected to reproduce and generate two offspring. The two offspring will replace the two solutions with the worst fitness from the tournament. The difference in the number of mating events rises from the number of simulated epidemics used to calculate fitness. The duration and spread fitness use a limited number of simulated epidemics, between 1 and 5, set by the programmer. This drastically increases the speed of the fitness evaluation but can result in a solution getting 'lucky' by achieving a fitness value that does not represent the actual quality of the network. Therefore, the number of mating events must be higher and a modified size-seven tournament selection is used, known as *skeptical* tournament selection. The skeptical part results in the fitness of the parents being recalculated after reproduction. Due to the low number of simulated epidemics used to determine fitness, a network may achieve an artificially high fitness due to the stochastic nature of epidemics. The re-calculation of fitness after being selected for reproduction means that a network is unlikely to repeatedly be selected unless it's fitness value represents the true quality of the network.

4.1.5 Reproduction

The two candidate solutions selected via tournament selection are labelled *parents*. These two parents are used to generate two *children*. This is done using two-point crossover by selecting two crossover points, CP_1 and CP_2, in the range $[1, 256]$. The first child receives the first CP_1 edge-operations from the first parent, edge-operations $(CP_1, CP_2]$ from the second parent, and the last $256 - CP_2$ edge-operations again from the first parent. The second child is created similarly: $[1, CP_1]$ from the second parent, (CP_1, CP_2) from the first, and $[CP_2, 256]$ from the second. An example of two-point crossover being applied to two chromosomes of length 10 is shown in Fig. 4.5. Next, the two children undergo mutation.

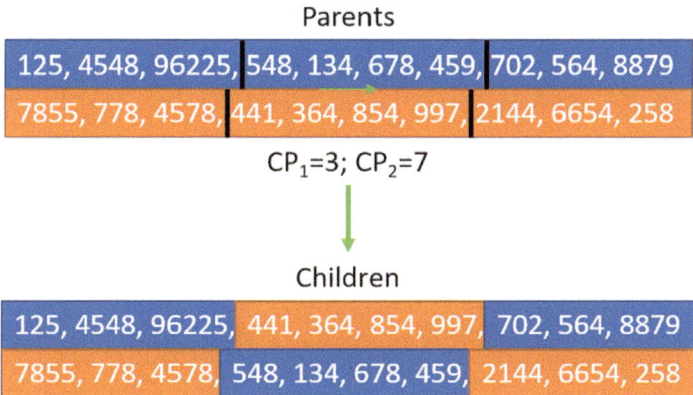

Fig. 4.5 And example of two-point crossover with crossover points $CP_1 = 3$ and $CP_2 = 7$ being applied to two parents, generating two children

4.1.6 Mutation

The two newly generated children solutions undergo 1–3 mutations, with the number of mutations being decided uniformly at random. Each mutation randomly replaces one edge-operation in the chromosome with a new operation selected at random according to the same probability distribution used during initialization. After mutation occurs these children undergo fitness evaluation and replace the two members of the tournament with the worst fitness.

4.1.7 Parameter Selection

There are several parameters for the system. A summary of their values is included in Table 4.2.

The parameter of the system yet to be defined is the edge-editing operation probability distribution. This distribution is itself comprised of nine densities representing the likelihood of each operation being selected. Though, since the densities must sum to one, it is considered only eight parameters as selecting eight determines the value of the ninth. This distribution impacts the results of the system as it directs what will occur with the edges in the network. For example, if a network with an abundance of edges results in an increased to fitness, then a high proportion of the operations must to be operations which add edges. Thus, it is important that the system be run with several probability distributions that adequately explore the different operations and their combinations. To demonstrate the difficulty of creating a set of densities to explore the potential parameter space, we investigate doing so with three densities which add to one, label them A, B, and C such that $A + B + C = 1.0$.

Table 4.2 The parameters used to run the system

Parameter	Value
Number of nodes	128
Initial network	Ring and PowerLaw cluster
Number of operations	256
Probability distribution	Several (read below)
α	0.50
Mating events	40 000 or 500 000
Fitness function	Profile matching, epidemic length, or spread
Simulated epidemics for fitness	50 or 1–5
Maximum number of mutations	3

Table 4.3 Probability distributions possible for three variable which sum to one, where A and B can be one of $\{0.10, 0.25, 0.50, 0.75, 0.90\}$

A	B	C
0.10	0.10	0.80
0.10	0.25	0.65
0.10	0.50	0.40
0.10	0.75	0.15
0.10	0.90	0.00
0.25	0.10	0.65
0.25	0.25	0.50
0.25	0.50	0.25
0.25	0.75	0.00
0.50	0.10	0.40
0.50	0.25	0.25
0.50	0.50	0.00
0.75	0.10	0.15
0.75	0.25	0.00
0.90	0.10	0.00

If the possible values of A and B are in the set $\{0.10, 0.25, 0.50, 0.75, 0.90\}$, then there would be 15 possible probability distributions, which are given in Table 4.3. Scaling this up to nine densities is not feasible. Thus, another method known as *point packing* was used to determine sets of densities used to run the system.

A point packing is itself an evolutionary algorithm which packs a parameter space with as many points as possible while respecting a user defined minimum spacing between points.

Therefore, each point in a packing is a probability distribution used to select edge operations to run the system. It has been shown that point packings are effective at thoroughly
exploring a parameter space for a problem (Ashlock and Graether 2016). This is done by
using far fewer parameter settings than was observed when a traditional parameter sweep
is conducted, like in Table 4.3. In addition, should a more thorough exploration be desired,
a researcher need only reduce the minimum distance between points. The underlying algorithm used to generate points in a point packing is Conway's Lexicode Algorithm, provided
in Algorithm 4.1.

Algorithm 4.1 Conway's Lexicode Algorithm

Inputs: a set S of points in some order, a minimum distance δ.
Output: a subset T of S with minimum distance δ.

1: Initialize T to be empty
2: **for all** $s \in S$ **do**
3:    **if** $\forall t \in T$: distance between s and $t \geq \delta$ **then**
4:       $T = T \cup \{s\}$
5:    **end if**
6: **end for**
7: Return(T)

The point packing evolutionary algorithm evolves a population of 4000 point packings. At
the end of evolution, the point packing with the largest number of points (parameter settings)
is selected to run the system. To run this algorithm, a researcher chooses a minimum distance
between the parameter settings, δ. The initial population of packings is generated, one-by-
one. First, randomly generate 1000 points in the parameter space and use this as the input
parameter S in Algorithm 4.1. The output is added to the population as one of the point
packings.

Evolutionary algorithms use crossover to capitalize on solutions that have the best fitness
while using mutation to introduce enough diversity to avoid locally maximal solutions. In
contrast, the evolutionary algorithm used to achieve a point packing with the most points uses
one variation operation–Conway Crossover Operator (CCO). This operator first selects two
collections of parameter settings and combines these sets into one set. From there, twenty
new points are generated randomly and they are added to the combined set. This set is then
shuffled, and a new collection of points obeying the minimum distance between points is
generated using Algorithm 4.1. This process accomplishes both crossover, by combining
two collections, and mutation, by introducing randomly generated PSs.

Each mating event randomly chooses three members of the population and the two with
the largest collection of points are subjected to CCO and the newly generated collection
replaces the collection with the least number of points. Thirty runs are conducted, each

comprised of 1 000 000 mating events. Though a single run would still result in a point packing of the space, repeating the experiment generally yields larger point packings than seen in a single run. The run that produces a collection with the most PSs is chosen for the experiment because if there are more points obeying the minimum distance in a set space then the space is the best explored using that largest collection of points.

4.2   Applying to Epidemic Data

4.2.1   Real Life Data

Real life data can be messy, and it isn't always in the exact form that you need. For this process, you need data that shows the number of new cases or number of deaths over time. The unit of time is not important, usually it is either days or weeks. In order to know the number of cases there must be some sort of test for the disease. This is not always available. For example, if you were interested in contact networks for the 1918 flu pandemic, the only data you would be able to get is the number of deaths per day. Sometimes the date of infection is hard to determine. For example, with the HIV/AIDS pandemic, the incubation period for the disease is very long, so the date of a positive test could be well after the date of infection. With the COVID-19 pandemic, on the other hand, the date of onset of symptoms is a good approximation of the date of infection.

Better results are obtained if you smooth the data first. For the COVID-19 pandemic, almost every health unit that published data made a bar graph of the number of cases per day and then showed a line graph with a 7-day moving average. That 7-day average could get you better results than the bar graph because it filters out irrelevant information like if no tests were done on a holiday or if there was a day when extra people were tested due to an outbreak.

Furthermore, real life data has other inaccuracies. It is often updated daily or even several times a day. Sometimes these updates change values in the past, especially if you're looking at date of onset of symptoms rather than date of test. There can be a need to protect privacy that results in some data being deleted or noise being added to the data.

It is important to be mindful of the scope of the data. You will get a very different contact network that can be interpreted in very different ways if you are looking at data for a small group of people, say a university community, versus a large community, say an entire country. With the small group, there may be contacts that expose people that are not included in the data. With the large group, your evolved contact network could well be missing constraints that exist in the real world, like the extent of cross country travel.

Another important consideration is how many nodes to include in the evolved contact network. The most direct choice is the number of people who got sick. Then, the contact network shows the way in which the disease was spread amongst them. This often works

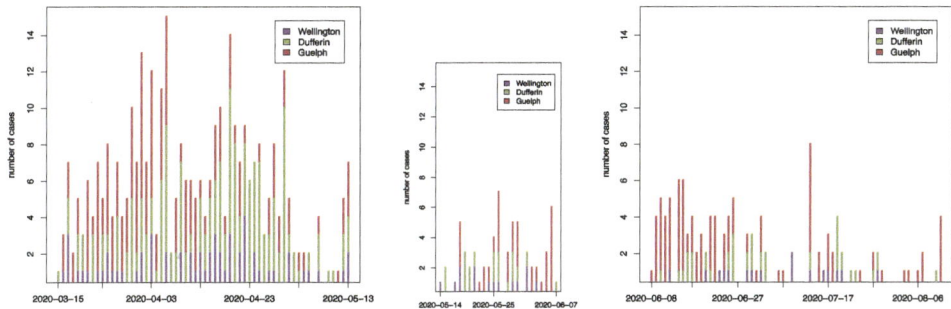

Fig. 4.6 Epidemic profiles for Wellington–Dufferin–Guelph Health Unit from Mar. 15 to Aug. 6, 2020

well. But, with any pandemic, there are cases that are never reported. So, sometimes there is value in adding some extra nodes to model that.

4.2.1.1 Wellington–Dufferin–Guelph Health Unit During COVID Pandemic

As an example of real life epidemic data, we present data from the Wellington–Dufferin–Guelph Health Unit in Ontario, Canada in Fig. 4.6.

4.3 Visualizations

The system is used to generate personal contact networks. These can be visualized in a number of ways. First, this can be done by generating images showing the nodes and the edges between said nodes. Two examples of this visualization can be seen in Figs. 4.7 and 4.8. Another way to visualize these networks, according to their performance, would be by demonstrating the curves generated by the epidemics which are simulated on the networks. This can be seen in Fig. 4.9.

4.3.1 Visualizing Evolved Networks

Contact networks that realistically represent a community in a real epidemic have too many nodes to be directly visualized. Our example data for the Wellington–Dufferin–Guelph Health Unit during the first wave of the COVID pandemic in the spring of 2020 is for a community of 272,000 people with 344 cases. Even if the evolved network only represents the infected people, it still has too many nodes to be able to represent it so that it can be made sense of easily. It is important to be able to do this, because the evolutionary algorithm

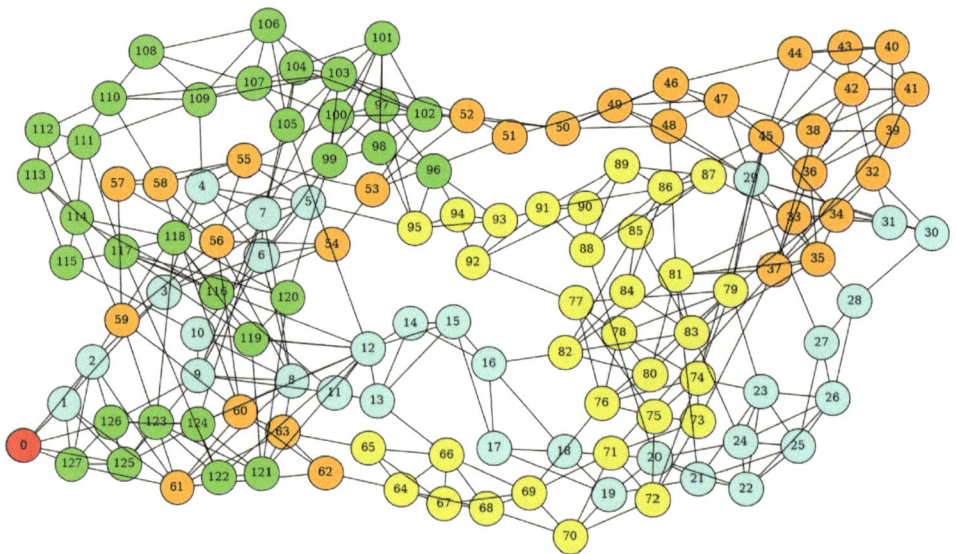

Fig. 4.7 A network with 128 nodes generated using the initial ring network and profile matching fitness on profile 2. The nodes are coloured by index, and patient zero is indicated in red

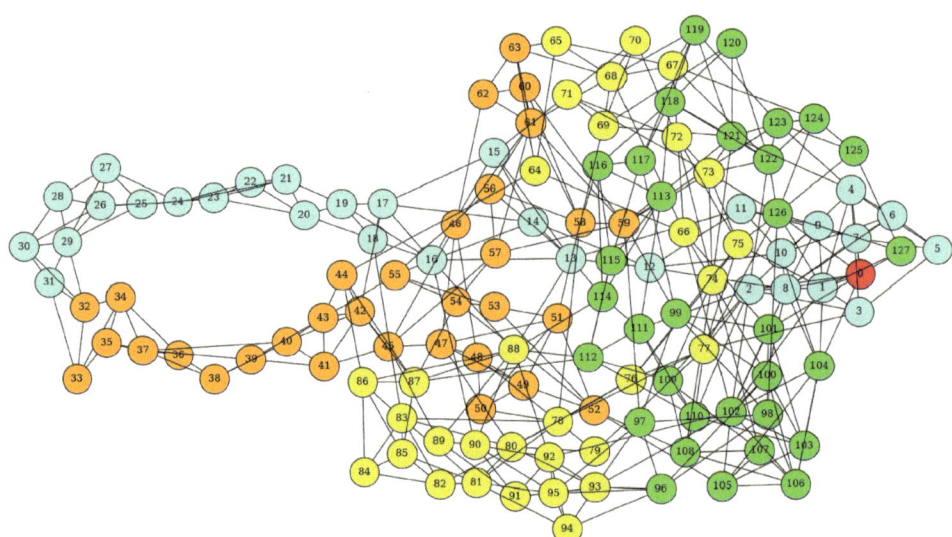

Fig. 4.8 A network with 128 nodes generated using the initial ring network and profile matching fitness on profile 2. The nodes are coloured by index, and patient zero is indicated in red

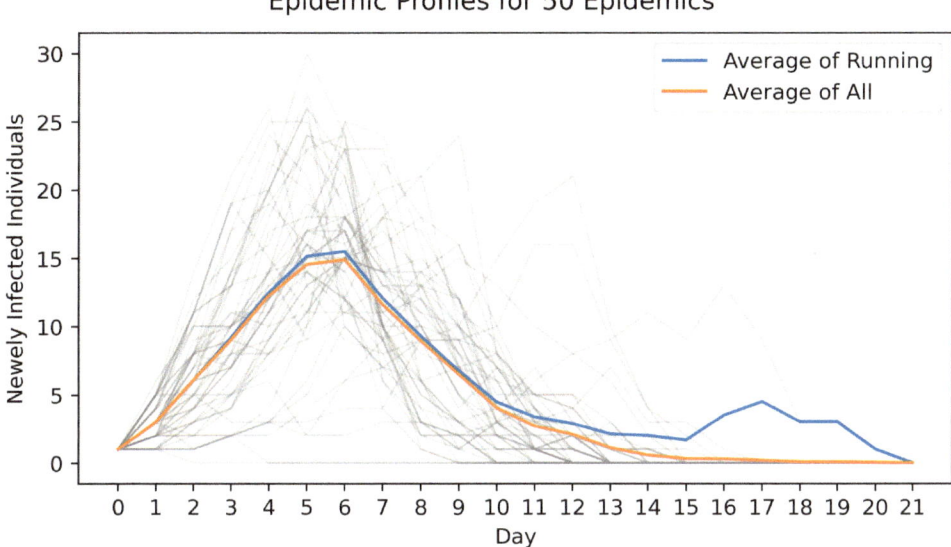

Fig. 4.9 The epidemic curves generated by 50 simulated epidemics on a network

will produce many possible matches to the epidemic profile. If public health officials want to use one of these networks to better understand the spread of the epidemic through the community, they need a way to pick the solution that is the best fit.

References

R. Albert, A.L. Barabasi, Statistical mechanics of complex networks. Rev. Modern Phys. **74**(1), 47–97 (2002)

D. Ashlock, S. Graether, Conway crossover to create hyperdimensional point packings, with applications, in *Proceedings of the 2016 Congress on Evolutionary Computation* (IEEE Press, Piscataway, NJ, 2016), pp. 1570–1577

C. Darwin, *The Origin of Species*. Five Foot Shelf of Books. P. F. Collier (1909). https://books.google.ca/books?id=YY4EAAAAYAAJ

D.J. Futuyma, M. Kirkpatrick, *Evolution* (Sinauer Associates, 2017)

V. Latora, A. Nyamba, J. Simpore, B. Sylvette, S. Diane, B. Sylvére, S. Musumeci, Network of sexual contacts and sexually transmitted hiv infection in burkina faso. J. Med. Virol. **78**(6), 724–729 (2006). https://doi.org/10.1002/jmv.20614

F. Liljeros, C.R. Edling, L.A. Nunes Amaral, H.E.Stanley, Y. Åberg, The web of human sexual contacts. Nature **411**(6840), 907–908 (2001). ISSN 1476-4687 https://doi.org/10.1038/35082140

S. Russell, P. Norvig, *Artificial Intelligence: A Modern Approach* (CreateSpace Independent Publishing Platform, 2016). ISBN 9781537600314. https://books.google.ca/books?id=PQI7vgAACAAJ

R. Vega Jimenez, M. Dubé, S. Houghten, J. Hughes, Weighting on the world to change... an epidemic, in *2021 IEEE Congress on Evolutionary Computation (CEC)* (2021), pp. 450–457. https://doi.org/10.1109/CEC45853.2021.9504685

Vaccine Distribution 5

At the time of writing, the system described within this chapter is considered a work in progress. It is entirely functional, has many features included, and is designed to be modular in order to make customization simple. However, the authors expect to continue expanding the system with multiple additional features. Current results are reported in Amin et al. (2021) and Hughes et al. (2020).

Regrettably, the state of the code leaves something to be desired. One of the goals the authors have is to refactor the system significantly to be more user friendly.

For the most up-to-date version of the system, visit the following GitHub page: https://github.com/convergencelab/eCov-GP.

Despite the state of the world during the first half of 2020, the SARS-CoV-2 vaccine was developed, approved, and deployed astonishingly quickly; plagued with resource, supply chain, policy, and morale issues, teams of scientists, engineers, and decision-makers achieved something that will be looked back on by optimists as evidence that we can, when push comes to shove, solve immediate complex problems.

5.1   How Best to Vaccinate a Population

When a limited supply of vaccines become available during a global pandemic, how best are they applied to a population such that the spread and impact of the disease is minimized?

Many jurisdictions implemented a phased vaccine rollout as a consequence of the limited global supply. It was common for these jurisdictions, at least in North America, to follow the Centers for Disease Control and Prevention (CDC) guidelines on prioritizing individuals

J. Hughes et al., *AI Versus Epidemics*, Synthesis Lectures on Learning, Networks, and Algorithms, https://doi.org/10.1007/978-3-031-64373-6_5

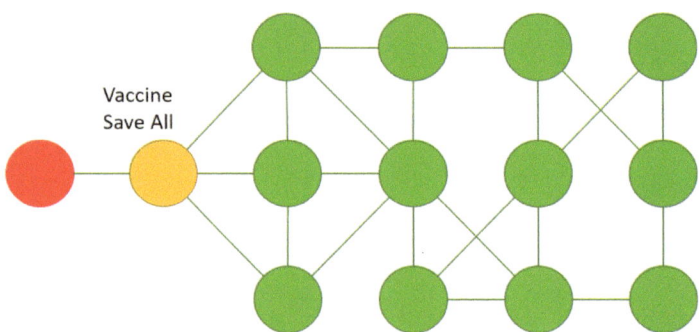

Fig. 5.1 An idealized scenario where a single vaccine can stop the spread of an infectious disease. The red node represents an individual that is infectious, while the green nodes are those that are susceptible to the disease. By vaccinating an individual intelligently (yellow node), the entire population is protected

for vaccines (Ahmed 2013; Smith 2010). Many considerations, such as risk analysis, health economics, implementation issues, and demographic information are used when determining priorities in order to best protect the population.

Focusing on at risk individuals and those under high viral loads, such as healthcare workers, has been critically important, and following CDC recommendations has been effective; however, a new type of analysis focusing on the topology and structure of social contact networks can augment decision making. By exploiting the features of a social contact network, it is possible to prioritize which individuals within a population to vaccinate[1] to limit, or stop, the spread of a disease through the network. Figure 5.1 provides an illustration of how intelligently applying vaccines to a population based on the structure of the social contact network can minimize the impact of the infectious disease on the community. Although this figure provides an idealized best case scenario, it demonstrates how a single vaccine can have a maximal impact.

One of the most related works was performed by Zhang et al. (2015) and Thakare and Mathurkar (2016). Although this work was done a few years before the COVID-19 pandemic, it is nevertheless relevant as it focuses on limiting the spread of an infections disease. The authors investigated vaccination strategies based on data from personal contact networks and compared them to a baseline strategy of a first come first served approach to vaccination. This first come first served approach is one of the baseline strategies we use as a comparison.

Dubé et al. (2020a) investigated multiple vaccination strategies and their impact on the duration and spread of a disease throughout a social contact network. Strategies investigated included measures such as the degree of a vertex, vaccinating all neighbours of infected individuals, and random (first come first served) vaccination strategies.

---

[1] Although "vaccinate" is used here, we make use of the term "mitigation strategy" throughout as the ideas are generalizable well beyond only vaccines.

Other related work from Ashlock (2020), Dubé et al. (2020a, b) and Timmins and Ashlock (2017) focused on the generation of graphs with evolutionary algorithms to match the spread of a disease based on known, real-world epidemic profiles.

Although this chapter discusses the application of mitigation strategies to a community during a pandemic, the system itself is generalizable beyond pandemics, and ultimately useful when analyzing the distribution of scarce resources.

Within this chapter, an explanation of how a graph can represent a social contact network for a given community is provided in Sects. 5.2, 5.2.1.4 and 5.4 discuss how an infectious disease scenario is simulated on the graphs. Although many forms of artificial intelligence and machine learning are applicable, Sect. 5.5 provides an explanation on how to make use of Genetic Programming (see Chap. 2) for the discovery of novel and effective vaccination strategies based on the graph topology. Finally, Sect. 5.6 presents interesting and noteworthy vaccination strategies found by our system. We chose to keep Sect. 5.6 discussion at a relatively high-level as not to overwhelm the reader with tables and tables of numbers as we feel that may distract from the key details. For a more in-depth discussion and analysis of results, refer to Hughes et al. (2020) and Amin et al. (2021) as they are the most recent published results at the time of writing.

5.2   Graphs as a Representation for Social Contact Networks

A graph/network, defined as a set of vertices/nodes representing individuals, and edges between vertices representing close enough contact between individuals for an infectious disease transmission, is a natural mathematical representation of a social contact network. Figure 5.2 provides a illustration of how a graph may represent social contact networks.

The graphs used within the system are implemented with *NetworkX*, a comprehensive Python package for graph creation and manipulation (Hagberg et al. 2008). The use of this package is ideal for our system for discovering vaccine strategies as it can work with any arbitrary graph, as long as it can be encoded as an adjacency list. This allows the user of our system to find vaccine strategies for specific social contact networks. For example, if a social contact network for a specific community is known, perhaps created based on cellphone or GPS data, then specialized vaccination strategies for that community could be created. Having such a graph would be important as there is evidence that the topology of the social contact network impacts the spread of an infectious disease (Da Gama and Nunes 2006; Keeling and Eames 2005).

Alternatively, given the difficulty of obtaining a graph representing an actual community, the system can generate and use random graphs for vaccination strategy discovery. Any method for generating a random graph could be incorporated into the system, but as of the time of writing, *Erdős–Rényi* (ER) (Erdős and Rényi 1959), *Newman–Watts–Strogatz* (NWS) (Newman and Watts 1999), *Barabási–Albert* (BA) (Barabási and Albert 1999), and *Powerlaw Cluster Graphs* (PCG) (Holme and Kim 2002) are included. Although ideally

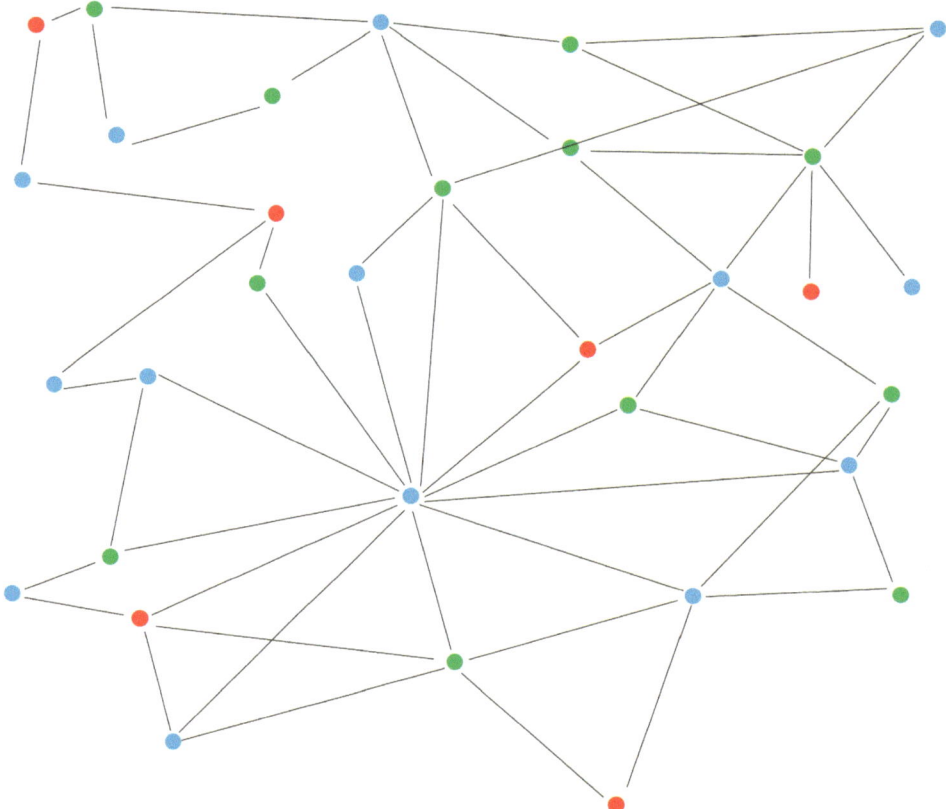

Fig. 5.2 A graph representation of a social contact network for a given population. Nodes/vertices represent individuals and edges represent a sufficiently close and consistent contact between individuals such that an infectious disease may spread from one to the other. This representation can easily be generalized to weighted graphs where weights represent the *closeness* of a given contact

one would want to evolve a strategy for a specific population's social contact network, these random graphs are effective at finding vaccine strategies that work well in general, regardless of the specific topology of the graph.

Each of the already included graph types have their advantages, but more recently the focus has been on the PCGs as they have small world properties (Watts and Strogatz 1998) and are scale-free, which is thought to better represent real social contact networks, although this is not universally accepted (Broido and Clauset 2019). Regardless, of the already included random graphs, the PCGs have been the primary graph type used within the system. Ultimately, however, the system is designed to be modular and, as already discussed, any arbitrary graph or graph generation strategy may be incorporated into the system.

When generating the graphs, regardless of their type, the settings used were selected such that they had similar values for various graph measures. Table 5.1 provides a view of the

Table 5.1 Values for the average powerlaw cluster graph used in much of the work. Some values are fixed, but due to the stochastic nature in which these graphs are generated, some values differ across individual graphs

Number of vertices	500
Average edge count	~1980
Min. degree	4
Avg. degree	~8
Max. degree	~(70 − 120)
Min. dist.	1
Avg. dist.	~3
Max. dist.	5
Min. clustering coef.	0
Avg. clustering coef.	~(0.31 − 0.33)
Max. clustering coef.	1

graph measure values used in previous work. Since each graph type has their own settings, no universally applied values were used other than the number of vertices. For example, with the PCGs, the number of edges was 500, the edges to add to a vertex was 4, and the probability to add a triangle was 66%. The values provided here are for illustrative purposes and should not be interpreted as being particularly relevant for any specific community.

Since the social contact networks are not static, especially over long periods of time, dynamic graphs—graphs that slowly alter their topology—were explored in Amin et al. (2021). Details on how the graphs were altered and how the alterations are parameterized are explained within the article; however, the major conclusion of the work was that there was no meaningful evidence that the use of dynamic graphs provided higher quality vaccination strategies when compared to static graphs.

5.2.1   Graph Measures

Various graph summary statistics and other measures of the current state of a simulated pandemic are used as the basis for decision making about which individuals to vaccinate at which time. For example, if a vertex has a particularly high degree and an infected neighbour, perhaps it would be wise to vaccinate that individual. For a more complex example, it may be prudent to vaccinate someone if they exist in the shortest path between many pairs of vertices. These graph measures are the parameters used by the vaccine decision making function—we consider the rules for considering an individual eligible for a vaccine a *function*.

A few graph summary statistics are included within Table 5.1, but many more are considered within the system and discussed below. These measures are broken into categories based on what and how they are calculated. Like most things within the system, the set of measures used is easy to change and add to. Many measures are self explanatory, but a brief description of the measures are included here.[2] Additional details on each measure, including specific algorithm names and computational complexity of the calculation, may be found in previous work (Amin et al. 2021; Hughes et al. 2020).

5.2.1.1 Static Measures

The static measures are those that only need to be calculated once before the start of any simulation. Most of these measures are quite computationally expensive, so it is fortunate that these measures can be stored for lookup.

- **Travelers**—Although *travelers* are not well defined by any means, they represent vertices within the graph that connect more densely connected clusters. There are many possible strategies for finding these travellers, but in our work the Clauset–Newman–Moore greedy modularity maximization algorithm Clauset et al. (2004) was used to identify communities and then the minimum edge cut was done to identify vertices connecting these communities. This produces a set of vertices. Figure 5.3 shows an example of travellers.
- **Average Degree**—The average degree of all vertices within the graph. This produces a single value.
- **Minimum Vertex Cover**—The approximation of which vertices are contained within the minimum vertex cover for the graph. This produces a set of vertices.
- **Average Shortest Distance**—The average shortest distance from all vertices to all other vertices. This is a single value.

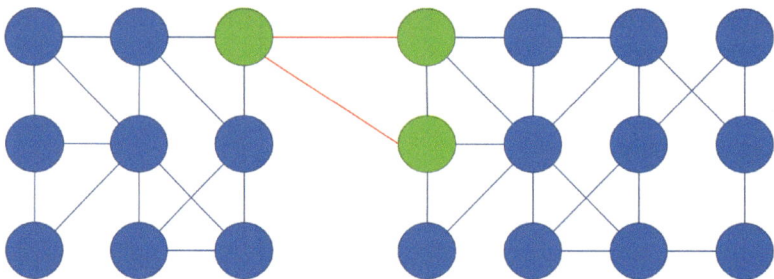

Fig. 5.3 Example of "travellers". Within this graph there are two closely connected communities, but there are only three vertices that connect the two communities. These individuals are considered the "travellers" as they *travel* between these communities

---

[2] If the reader feels overwhelmed by the number of measures and their descriptions, feel free to skip the next sections. The main point being communicated is that various graph measures and summary statistics can be calculated and used for decision making.

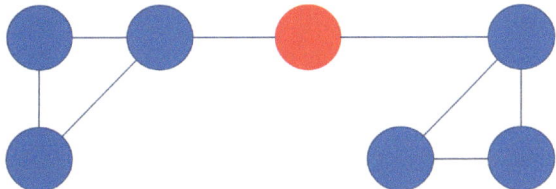

Fig. 5.4 Depiction of the shortest path count. The vertex in the centre exists in 9 of the shortest paths within that graph. Although this is an extreme example, it demonstrates that the shortest path count provides a quick idea of how *important* that vertex is

- **Shortest Distance: All to All**—The shortest distance from all vertices to all other vertices. This generates a matrix.
- **Average Shortest Distance: One to All**—The average shortest distance a given vertex has from all other vertices. This generates a single value for each vertex.
- **Shortest Paths: All to All**—The shortest paths from all vertices to all other vertices. This generates a matrix of paths.
- **Shortest Path Count**—The number of times a given vertex exists within the shortest path from all possible pairs of any two vertices. This generates a single value for each vertex. Figure 5.4 shows an example of this measure.
- **Page Rank**—The Page Rank vertex weights, which provides a measure for the traffic through a node. This produces a single value for each vertex.
- **Clustering Coefficient**—The clustering coefficient of each vertex. This produces a single value for each vertex.

5.2.1.2 Global Measures
Global measures are those about the graph as a whole. These need to be calculated before every calculation of which vertices should receive a vaccine.

- **Number of Vertices in a Given State**—The count of vertices in a particular pandemic simulation state. For example, number of susceptible or infectious individuals. More details on the various states are discussed in Sect. 5.2.1.4. This provides a single value for each possible states.
- **Average Distance Between Vertices of a Given State**—The average distance between vertices of a pandemic simulation state. Similar to above, this could be the average distance between infectious individuals. This gives a single value for each possible state.

5.2.1.3 Local Measures

Local measures are those pertaining to an individual vertex, or a relatively small localized cluster of vertices.

- **Vertex Status**—The current state of an individual vertex. The various states are discussed within Sect. 5.2.1.4. Produces a single value.
- **Vertex Degree**—The degree/number of neighbours an individual vertex has. Produces a single value.
- **Average Neighbour Degree**—The average degree/number of neighbours each neighbour of the individual vertex has. Produces a single value.
- **Neighbours of a Given State**—The number of neighbours an individual vertex has of a given state. For example, the number of infectious neighbours. Produces a single value.
- **Is Traveler**—A Boolean specifying if the vertex is contained within the traveller set described in Sect. 5.2.1.1.
- **In Minimum Vertex Cover**—A Boolean specifying if a vertex is contained within the approximated minimal vertex cover. The approximated minimum vertex cover was calculated as a static measure described in Sect. 5.2.1.1.
- **Shortest Distance to a Vertex of a Given State**—The shortest path length to closest vertex of a given state. This returns a single value.
- **Vertex Average Distance**—The average distance the specified individual has to all other vertices. This value was calculated as one of the static measures described in Sect. 5.2.1.1.
- **Shortest Path Count**—The number of times the vertex exists within the shortest path between any two vertices. This value was calculated as one of the static measures described in Sect. 5.2.1.1.
- **Vertex Page Rank Weight**—The page rank weight of the vertex as calculated by the static measure described in Sect. 5.2.1.1.
- **Vertex Clustering Coefficient**—The vertex's clustering coefficient as calculated by the static measure described in Sect. 5.2.1.1.

5.2.1.4 Extra Measures

- **Mitigation Count**—The number of remaining mitigations (e.g., vaccines) available. Details on how the number of vaccines available impact the simulation are described in Sect. 5.4.
- **Is Mitigation Available**—A Boolean indicating if any mitigations are remaining for a vaccination period. This measure is related to *mitigation count* and is TRUE if the number of mitigations remaining is greater than 0.
- **Simulation Step**—The current step of the simulation. Details on the simulation are presented in Sect. 5.4. This returns a single value.

5.3   The SEIR Model of an Infectious Disease

There are many mathematical epidemic models available for simulating the spread of an infectious disease, with many being based on the Susceptible-Infectious-Removed (SIR) model (Kermack and McKendrick 1927). Within the SIR model, individuals are either *susceptible* to the disease, meaning they may become infected, *infectious*, meaning they are capable of spreading the disease, or *removed*, meaning they are no longer able to spread the disease and, based on this model, are not able to become infected again. The SIR model is simple to use for simulating an infectious disease scenario—all individuals within a simulation fall into one of the three sets—susceptible (S), infectious (I), and removed (R)—with a probability to transition from S $\rightarrow$ I, and another probability to transition from I $\rightarrow$ R.

Here we make use of the Susceptible-Exposed-Infectious-Removed (SEIR) model (Aron and Schwartz 1984), which is based on the SIR model, but includes a fourth set, *exposed* (E), which means the individual has been exposed to the disease, but has yet to become infectious. This alters the state transitions to become S $\rightarrow$ E, E $\rightarrow$ I, and I $\rightarrow$ R.

Hence looking at the rates of transmission between states, α, β, and γ, we come to the following equation:

$$S \underset{\beta}{\rightarrow} E \underset{\alpha}{\rightarrow} I \underset{\gamma}{\rightarrow} R \tag{5.1}$$

The system is designed to work with arbitrary epidemic models, but the choice of the SEIR model for the work with COVID-19 was due to the disease's long incubation period. Recently, the SEIR model has been popular in modelling SARS-CoV-2 within the relevant literature (Prem et al. 2020). There are shortcomings with the model for SARS-CoV-2, such as presymptomatic and asymptomatic individuals being infectious (Furukawa et al. 2020); however, the authors remind the reader that modality was an important design decision for the system and the choice of infectious disease model and parameters can be switched out for another model relatively simply.

Here we provide the parameter values used in our previous work. Although these values were selected based on what was reported within the literature on SARS-CoV-2 (Prem et al. 2020), they should not be considered to be authoritative as the values may differ significantly between communities and the particular strain of the disease (He et al. 2020; Wang et al. 2020; Woelfel et al. 2020). Further, this system is more generally applicable to other infectious diseases, and as with most other values discussed within this Chapter, they are parameters that can be adjusted as needed by the users. The simulations were run with each individual within the graph having a 2% chance of starting within the infectious state (referred to as I_0), a probability of infecting, which controls the transition from S $\rightarrow$ E, of 9% (referred to as β), an incubation period of 6.4, controlling the transition from E $\rightarrow$ I of 6.4 (α), and a probability of recovering, controlling I $\rightarrow$ R, of 0.1333 (γ), and a probability.

The Python library, *Network Diffusion Library* (NDLib) was used for simulating the epidemics in this work (Rossetti et al. 2017, 2018). NDLib provides a suite of models and various other tools to aid in the study of diffusion processes within complex networks. It also includes mechanisms for defining custom models for a deeper analysis into nuanced questions. Beyond a comprehensive set of tools for studying infectious diseases, it includes models for studying opinion dynamics. The library is built on and integrates well with NetworkX, enabling the use of many existing graph algorithms (Hagberg et al. 2008), which was critically important as many of the graph measures discussed in Sect. 5.2.1 made use of the library's functionality.

5.4   Simulating an Infectious Disease Scenario with Interventions

A whole simulation of an infectious disease scenario is needed to evaluate the effectiveness of a given intervention strategy. The high-level strategy is to run the given epidemic model, which in our case is the SEIR model, for some set number of iterations.

In our work, the number of iterations is considered the number of days the simulation, which is parameterized and should be chosen such that the epidemic model has an opportunity to complete and no more disease is spreading throughout the network. The exact number of days selected will depend on the size of the graph, how connected the graph is, and the specific parameters for the given infectious disease model. In our experiments, the number of days ranged from 98 to 140.

When work began on this project, vaccines for SARS-CoV-2 were expected not to be available for some time. Further, the amount of vaccines that would be available, when made available, was assumed to be low as many jurisdictions would be competing to obtain vaccines for their populations. For these reasons, our experiments only made vaccines available periodically throughout the simulation, and when they were available, a restricted amount was available. We used a 7 day interval (once per week) and only made 30 vaccines available. Again, these values are parameterized and can be altered to suit the user's needs.

On a given day that vaccines were available, the population of susceptible and exposed individuals were candidates for vaccination; although we are omnipotent in our simulation and know the difference between susceptible and exposed, we assume that the individuals within the simulation would not know the difference between a susceptible and exposed since exposed individuals present no symptoms. The susceptible and exposed individuals were shuffled to provide a first-come-first-served scenario, and if (a) the individual met the criteria for a vaccine (the vaccination strategy being evolved, described in Sect. 5.5) (e.g., has a degree greater than 5), and (b) there are vaccines currently available, then the individual received the vaccine.

In our simulations, when a susceptible individual received a vaccine, they would transition from S $\rightarrow$ R, meaning they are not unable to contract or spread the disease. However, if it was the case that the individual was exposed and not susceptible, the vaccine would have no effect and the individual would remain in the exposed set, thereby wasting a vaccine.

It is important to emphasize that, although our work focused on the intervention/mitigation for the infectious disease being vaccines, the intervention could be any mechanism having any affect on the spread of the disease. In our experiments, we considered vaccines having the effect of transitioning the individual to the removed set, but there was nothing preventing us from including, for example, a vaccine efficacy rate. Another reasonable alternative could be, for example, treating the intervention as masking and the masks having the effect of lowering the spread probability.

Additional flags were included in the system, such as *rollover* and *use all*, but were ultimately not used in any experiments. The idea of rollover was that, if it was the case that not all the vaccines were used on a given day, they would be added to the total vaccines made available on the next day vaccines were available. Use all was included to force the use of all vaccines, even if an individual did not meet the vaccine strategy's requirements. The purpose of including their description here is to emphasize that the system we have created is not ridged. Instead, it is a loose set of ideas that are designed to be altered as needed.

We performed simulations on both static and dynamic graphs—graphs that changed their topology throughout the simulation. The rate and how the topology changed was, like everything, parameterized and can be tuned to the user's needs.

Algorithm 5.1 presents the high-level algorithm for the simulations.

5.5   Genetic Programming for Finding Vaccination Strategies

In our work, evolutionary computation, or more precisely, genetic programming, was the algorithm used to discover/create vaccination strategies; however, the general ideas used for the overall system is applicable to many other forms of learning algorithms. Regardless of the algorithm used, a simulation of the infectious disease scenario, as discussed in Sect. 5.4, is used to measure a given vaccination strategy's *goodness*.

There are a number of reasons genetic programming is ideal for this problem, but two noteworthy features are (a) the final result is a human interpretable "program", and (b) given the population based search, a large suite of high-quality solutions are produced after a single run of the evolutionary search.

The programs being evolved by genetic programming are the vaccination strategies themselves. These programs are comprised of the graph measures discussed in Sect. 5.2.1, along with constant values within some pre-defined range, and various arithmetic, comparison, and logical operators (an example set of operators is presented in Table 5.2, but the language provided to the genetic programming system is parameterized and up to the users). The vaccination strategies being evolved can be as simple as vaccinate if the number of neighbours is greater than some value (e.g., $degree > 5$), or complex sets of rules containing if statements. Various example final vaccination strategies are presented in Sect. 5.6.

As mentioned above, in order to evaluate a single vaccination strategy, an entire simulation of the infectious disease scenario needs to take place. Although the settings used for the

---

Algorithm 5.1 High-level algorithm for the infectious disease with intervention simulations.

Input :
f: Function defining a mitigation strategy.
$ITERS$: Number of days the simulation lasts
$MEAS$: Graph measure and mitigation frequency
$MITS$: Number of mitigations available
Output :
If an individual is to be vaccinated (Boolean)

```
 1: for i ← 0 to ITERS do
 2:    // If Mitigation Day
 3:    if i ! = 0 and i % MEAS == 0 then
 4:       mits_used ← 0
 5:       susexp ← get_susceptible_exposed()
 6:       susexp ← shuffle(susexp)
 7:       m_global ← global_measures()
 8:       for all v ∈ susexp do
 9:          // If Mitigation Available
10:          if mits_used < MITS then
11:             m_local ← local_measures()
12:             m_extra ← extra_measures()
13:             // If Function Says Mitigate
14:             if f(m_global, m_local, m_extra) then
15:                // If Effective
16:                if status(v) is susceptible then
17:                   set_removed(v)
18:                end if
19:                mits_used ← mits_used + 1
20:             end if
21:          end if
22:       end for
23:    end if
24: end for
```

---

genetic programming system are up to the user (see Hughes et al. 2020 and Amin et al. 2021 for our specific settings), to provide a sense of the number of simulations needed in total, consider a population size of 1,000 running for 500 generations. Further, to provide statistical significance for any system wide analysis and to increase the chance of finding a particularly effective strategy, every experiment was repeated 100 times. This would result in a total of 50,000,000 simulations of an infectious disease. Fortunately this is computationally tractable on today's computers, but it does limit the size of the graphs on which the simulations are being performed.

Table 5.2 The "language" used for the genetic programming system used. In addition to the operators and constant values shown here, the graph measures discussed in Sect. 5.2.1. Details on genetic programming languages can be found in Sect. 2.4

Language	
Arithmetic operators	+
	−
	×
	÷ (protected)
Boolean operators	and
	or
	not
Comparison and conditional	>
	<
	==
	If, Then, Else
Constants/terminals	TRUE/FALSE
	Integers 0–30

The simulation is reset after every fitness evaluation, however the topology of the graph stays the same; only the initial conditions are changed. The topology remained the same for two main reasons—(a) re-evaluating all the static graph measures on a new topology every time was not feasible, and (b) one would not change the topology of the graph if they were searching for vaccination strategies for a specified graph topology, which is an important feature of the system (loading in a graph from an adjacency list). However, like everything else in the system, this is changeable and there is nothing stopping someone from generating new topologies every time. The value of changing the topology every time would be to ensure the vaccination strategies being evolved are strong in general, regardless of the topology, but the computational cost is currently too high and altering the initial conditions still yielded reasonably general vaccination strategies.

The evolutionary search is considered the "training" phase, and after the evolutionary algorithm is run, all vaccination strategies within the final population are "validated". The validation process consists of running the strategies on some number of different graph topologies for the purpose of ensuring the strategies are effective in general and not just a specific topology. In our experiments 50 graphs were used, but this can be scaled up or down as needed. Additionally, the validation step, as it is currently used, is not necessary if a specific graph topology was provided to the system.

After validation, some number of the best performing strategies are selected for testing. Testing is done on some number of graphs (we used 100) and their final results are used for comparison to one another and some basic vaccination strategies—strategies that were not developed by the system, but something a human may come up with (e.g., vaccinate high degree nodes). Depending on the user's needs, testing can be done on many runs on a single topology or a new topology for every test.

Once all testing results are compiled, they are compared to one another and investigated further.

5.6   Generated Strategies

Only a high-level summary view of the results are presented here. For a full analysis of results, please refer to the works in Hughes et al. (2020) and Amin et al. (2021). Only a few sets of numbers are presented as the high-level view should be sufficient to gain an understanding of what the results look like, how they can be interpreted, and how they impact the outcome of an infectious disease scenario. Including the full analysis may distract from the *meaning* of the results and the overall idea of using artificial intelligence to provide decision making on a graph.

The final vaccination strategies are represented as trees called "S-expressions", or, symbolic expressions, that ultimately represent a program. Figure 5.5 provides an example S-expression of a potential vaccination strategy. The displayed S-expression is not one that was developed by any of the experiments, but is entirely possible to be created by the system. This S-expression could be represented as an algorithm as seen in Algorithm 5.2.

The earlier strategies generated, which were presented in Hughes et al. (2020), were relatively simple since, at the time, fewer graph measures were included within the system. As additional measures were included, the complexity of the vaccination strategies grew, like those presented in Amin et al. (2021).

Some of the original, simpler strategies were as straightforward as $NB\_INF > 1$, or, if the number of infectious neighbours an individual has is greater than one, then vaccinate that individual. This strategy, although simple, is intuitive since it would make sense to vaccinate individuals that come into contact with those that are infectious.

Fig. 5.5 Example of a possible vaccination strategy evolved by the genetic programming system. This specific example says to vaccinate an individual if the number of neighbours they have infected is greater than 5 and the total number of infected individuals within the simulation is greater than 200

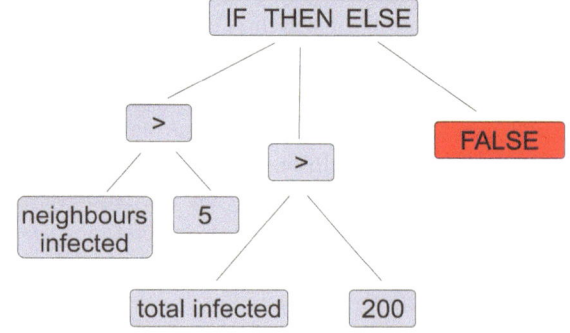

Algorithm 5.2 High-level algorithm for the infectious disease with intervention simulations.

Input : Various Graph Measures
Output : If an individual is to be vaccinated (Boolean)

1: **if** NUMBER_NEIGHBOURS_INFECTED > 5 **then**
2:    **return** TOTAL_INFECTED > 200
3: **else**
4:    **return** FALSE
5: **end if**

Another relatively simple strategy generated was $DEG > 10$ and $NB\_INF > 3$, or, if the number of neighbours an individual has is greater than 10, *and* the number of neighbours infectious is greater than three, then vaccinate. Again, simple and intuitive, but a little different when compared to the first. All intuition explanations of why a given strategy is effective is post hoc, thus they are at best hypotheses, however, they are all empirically analyzed (see Hughes et al. 2020). Where the first strategy was somewhat *aggressive* in vaccinating individuals, in the case of this second strategy, it seems more hesitant to apply a vaccine to an individual. Perhaps the evolutionary search found that, in order to preserve vaccines, it is better to vaccinate people who are in contact with infectious individuals *only* if they have a higher likelihood of spreading the disease broadly by being a high-degree node (having many contacts). This is reasonable given the constrained number of vaccines made available during the simulations—given the limited supply, it is better to apply vaccines where they will have the highest chance of minimizing/stopping the spread of the disease. Remember, for better or worse, in this public health scenario the goal is to protect the whole population as opposed to individuals.

The most complex vaccination strategy developed in the early work was IS_TRAV or $((14 - NB\_INF) < (DEG - 8))$, or, to slightly reorganize the expression with basic algebra, IS_TRAV or $(NB\_INF > (22 - DEG))$. This can be explained as, vaccinate if the individual is a "traveller" (connects communities of nodes) *or* if the neighbours infectious is greater than 22 minus the degree of the node. Although the "traveller" portion of the vaccination strategy makes sense, the other portion is difficult to wrap one's head around. Again, although we cannot truly know *why* the evolutionary search developed this strategy, we suggest that it has attempted to manage the degree requirement of the individual with the number of infectious neighbours. Consider Fig. 5.6 which shows the values required for an individual to be considered eligible for a vaccine. The lines intersect at 11, and for simplicity in the description, consider the inequality was greater than and equal to instead of just greater than. This means that, if someone has a degree of 11 and all 11 are infectious, then they should be vaccinated. However, as the degree of the individual grows, the number of infectious neighbours required before they are eligible for a vaccine becomes smaller. What makes this strategy interesting is that, like the previous strategy, it is more restrictive

Fig. 5.6 Plot showing the admissible values for an individual to be vaccinated according to $(NB\_INF > (22 - DEG))$. Note that the upper bound in this plot corresponds to the degree of the graph; the number of infected neighbours cannot exceed the number of neighbours

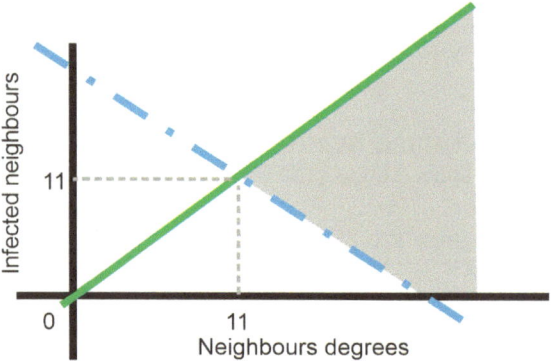

in who is eligible for a vaccine, but it has found a way for the vaccination strategy to become dynamic.

As the number and sophistication of the graph measures used increased, so did the complexity of the vaccination strategies found by the evolutionary search. Although a number of high-quality strategies were found and reported on by Amin et al. (2021), Algorithm 5.3 presents the top performing strategy found. As one can see, the complexity of the strategy is greater than those previously discussed. Our best attempt to describe why this strategy performs well is, *if* the individual is within the graph's approximate minimal vertex cover, then the value of d will be high *if* the individual is within many of the shortest paths between vertices (the value of the clustering coefficient will be negligible since it is a value between 0 and 1). If the individual is not within the minimal vertex cover, d will be large when they have many infected neighbours and/or the simulation is near the end when the number of removed individuals is high. Finally, given that fewer individuals will be susceptible or exposed as the simulation progresses, g will be large if the vertex has a large clustering coefficient.

The description of the algorithm is by no means simple, but the intuition is to vaccinate individuals deemed more important based on the graph centrality measures (e.g., clustering coefficient, minimal vertex cover, and frequency within the shortest paths between nodes), and as the simulation progresses, start vaccinating individuals more liberally.

Figures 5.7 and 5.8 show how the average cumulative total infected and average current infected curves differ under different circumstances. In both, the blue line shows what the curve looks like if no vaccines are used, the orange line is an indiscriminate first-come-first-served vaccination strategy, and the green line shows the curve of the evolved vaccination strategy presented in Algorithm 5.3. One can clearly see the impact of an effective vaccination strategy on the outcome of an infectious disease scenario.

When comparing the total infected numbers, as seen in Fig. 5.7, the median total infectious (which is the sum of all infected individuals over all days—e.g., individuals infections over a 7 day period would contribute 7 to the total) over 100 simulations with no vaccination strategy was 3565.0 ± 137.88. With an indiscriminate first-come-first-served vaccination

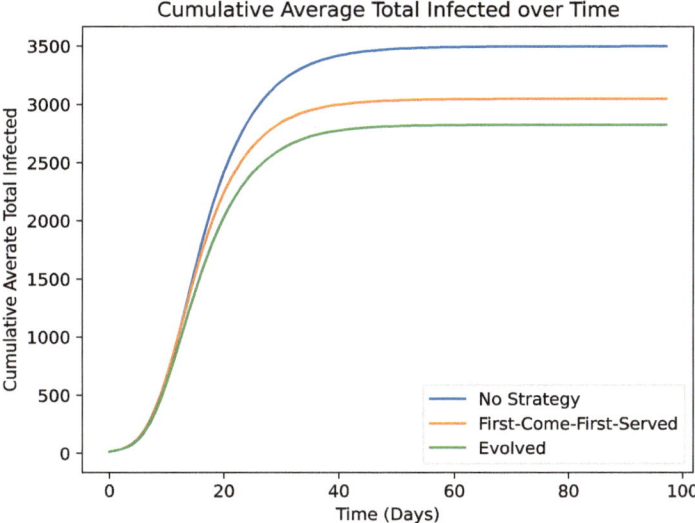

Fig. 5.7 Average cumulative total number of infected individuals over each day. Note that individuals are counted for each day they are infected. Observe that the use of vaccines has an impact, even if no systematic approach to vaccination is used. However, one can see that an evolved strategy improve the results while also using fewer vaccines

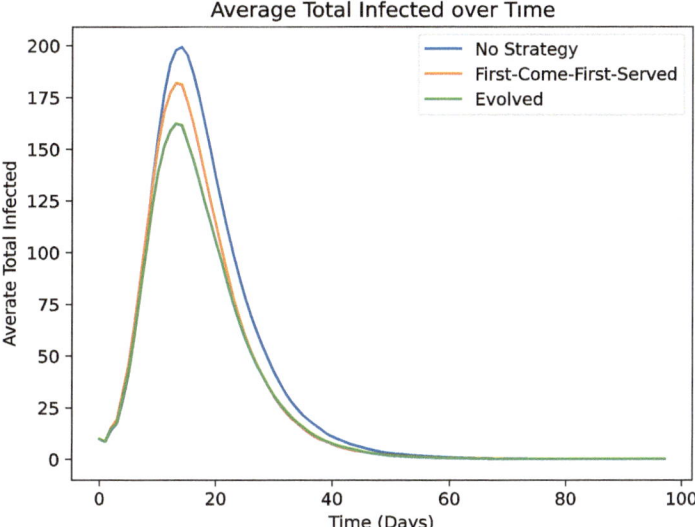

Fig. 5.8 Average total infected curves. Like Fig. 5.7, one can observe that the evolved strategy performs the best. Interestingly the curve is not so much "flattened" as it is just made smaller; there was no prolonged large number of infections occurring after the peak with the evolved strategy

---

Algorithm 5.3 Evolved Strategy.

Input : Various Graph Measures
Output : If an individual is to be vaccinated (Boolean)

1: **if** MINIMAL_VERTEX_COVER **then**
2:    d ← SHORTEST_PATH_COUNT + CLUSTERING_COEF
3: **else**
4:    d ← NUMBER_REMOVED × NEIGHBOURS_INFECTED
5: **end if**
6: g ← 4 × AVG_DEGREE × NUMBER_SUSEXP × CLUSTERING_COEF
7: Return $d > g$

---

strategy had 3049.6 ± 123.62, and the evolved strategy presented in Algorithm 5.3 had a total infected of 2797.5 ± 146.

Similarly, the maximum infected at any given time, as seen in Fig. 5.8, was 209.0 ± 10.25 for no vaccinations, 189.5 ± 10.75 for the indiscriminate first-come-first-served strategy, and 167.5 ± 15.25 for the evolved strategy.

As previously mentioned, a full analysis is presented in Hughes et al. (2020) and Amin et al. (2021). What is presented here is a high-level view of the system, how it it works, what the vaccination strategies look like, and the effectiveness of the evolved strategies for minimizing the impact of an infectious disease on a social network.

The takeaway is not the exact results presented here, but that the system exists and is heavily parameterized for general use. Further, the system can generate high-quality vaccination strategies that significantly outperform random or simple, human developed vaccination strategies; no one would have discovered the intricate evolved strategies on their own.

The authors consider that the software is still a work in progress as it will continually be enhanced—at the time of writing, the inclusion of age and comorbidity on vertices and their impact on vaccination strategies evolved.

References

F. Ahmed, U.S. advisory committee on immunization practices handbook for developing evidence-based recommendations. Technical Report, Centre for Disease Control and Prevention (2013). https://www.cdc.gov/vaccines/acip/recs/grade/downloads/handbook.pdf

S. Amin, S. Houghten, J.A. Hughes, Vaccinating a population is a changing programming problem, in *2021 IEEE Conference on Computational Intelligence in Bioinformatics and Computational Biology (CIBCB)* (IEEE, 2021), pp. 01–10

J.L. Aron, I.B. Schwartz, Seasonality and period-doubling bifurcations in an epidemic model. J. Theor. Biol. **110**(4), 665–679 (1984)

W. Ashlock, Visualizing contact networks evolved to fit epidemic profiles, in *2020 IEEE Conference on Computational Intelligence in Bioinformatics and Computational Biology (CIBCB)* (IEEE, 2020), pp. 1–8

A.-L. Barabási, R. Albert, Emergence of scaling in random networks. Science **286**(5439), 509–512 (1999)

A.D. Broido, A. Clauset, Scale-free networks are rare. Nat. Commun. **10**(1), 1–10 (2019)

A. Clauset, M.E.J. Newman, C. Moore, Finding community structure in very large networks. Phys. Rev. E **70**(6), 066111 (2004)

M.M.T. Da Gama, A. Nunes, Epidemics in small world networks. Eur. Phys. J. B-Condens. Matter Complex Syst. **50**(1–2), 205–208 (2006)

M. Dubé, S. Houghten, D. Ashlock, Modelling of vaccination strategies for epidemics using evolutionary computation, in *2020 IEEE Congress on Evolutionary Computation* (IEEE, 2020a)

M. Dubé, S. Houghten, D. Ashlock, J.A. Hughes, Evolving the curve, in *2020 IEEE Conference on Computational Intelligence in Bioinformatics and Computational Biology (CIBCB)* (IEEE, 2020b), pp. 1–8

P. Erdős, A. Rényi, On random graphs i. Publ. Math. Debrecen **6**(290–297), 18 (1959)

N.W. Furukawa, J.T. Brooks, J. Sobel, Evidence supporting transmission of severe acute respiratory syndrome coronavirus 2 while presymptomatic or asymptomatic. Emerg. Infect. Dis. **26**(7) (2020)

A. Hagberg, P. Swart, D.S. Chult, Exploring network structure, dynamics, and function using networkx. Technical Report, Los Alamos National Lab (LANL), Los Alamos, NM (United States) (2008)

X. He, E.H.Y. Lau, P. Wu, X. Deng, J. Wang, X. Hao, Y.C. Lau, J.Y. Wong, Y. Guan, X. Tan et al., Temporal dynamics in viral shedding and transmissibility of covid-19. Nat. Med. **26**(5), 672–675 (2020)

P. Holme, B.J. Kim, Growing scale-free networks with tunable clustering. Phys. Rev. E **65**(2), 026107 (2002)

J.A. Hughes, M. Dubé, S. Houghten, D. Ashlock, Vaccinating a population is a programming problem, in *2020 IEEE Conference on Computational Intelligence in Bioinformatics and Computational Biology (CIBCB)* (IEEE, 2020), pp. 1–8

M.J. Keeling, K.T.D. Eames, Networks and epidemic models. J. R. Soc. Interface **2**(4), 295–307 (2005)

W.O. Kermack, A.G. McKendrick, A contribution to the mathematical theory of epidemics. Proc. R. Soc. Lond. Ser. A (Containing papers of a Mathematical and Physical Character) **115**(772), 700–721 (1927)

M.E.J. Newman, D.J. Watts, Renormalization group analysis of the small-world network model. Phys. Lett. A **263**(4–6), 341–346 (1999)

K. Prem, Y. Liu, T.W. Russell, A.J. Kucharski, R.M. Eggo, N. Davies, S. Flasche, S. Clifford, C.A.B. Pearson, J.D. Munday et al., The effect of control strategies to reduce social mixing on outcomes of the covid-19 epidemic in Wuhan, China: a modelling study. The Lancet Public Health (2020)

G. Rossetti, L. Milli, S. Rinzivillo, A. Sirbu, D. Pedreschi, F. Giannotti, Ndlib: studying network diffusion dynamics, in *2017 IEEE International Conference on Data Science and Advanced Analytics (DSAA)* (IEEE, 2017), pp. 155–164

G. Rossetti, L. Milli, S. Rinzivillo, A. Sîrbu, D. Pedreschi, F. Giannotti, Ndlib: a python library to model and analyze diffusion processes over complex networks. Int. J. Data Sci. Anal. **5**(1), 61–79 (2018)

J.C. Smith, The structure, role, and procedures of the us advisory committee on immunization practices (acip). Vaccine **28**, A68–A75 (2010)

P.R. Thakare, S.S. Mathurkar, Modeling of epidemic spread by social interactions, in *2016 IEEE International Conference on Recent Trends in Electronics, Information & Communication Technology (RTEICT)* (IEEE, 2016), pp. 1320–1324

M. Timmins, D. Ashlock, Network induction for epidemic profiles with a novel representation. Biosystems **162**, 205–214 (2017)

D. Wang, H. Bo, H. Chang, F. Zhu, X. Liu, J. Zhang, B. Wang, H. Xiang, Z. Cheng, Y. Xiong et al., Clinical characteristics of 138 hospitalized patients with 2019 novel coronavirus-infected pneumonia in Wuhan, China. Jama **323**(11), 1061–1069 (2020)

D.J. Watts, S.H. Strogatz, Collective dynamics of 'small-world' networks. Nature **393**(6684), 440–442 (1998)

R. Woelfel et al., Clinical presentation and virological assessment of hospitalized cases of coronavirus disease 2019 in a travel-associated transmission cluster. MedRxiv (2020)

Z. Zhang, H. Wang, C. Wang, H. Fang, Modeling epidemics spreading on social contact networks. IEEE Trans. Emerg. Topics Comput. **3**(3), 410–419 (2015)

In working with our evolutionary algorithm for network induction and applying it to actual data, several issues arose. The first is that the search space of networks is enormous. The number of networks with n vertices is proportional to 2^{n^2}; it is hyper-exponential in the number of people infected. For real data, n is often quite large. In addition to the sheer size, these networks are made of arbitrarily labelled nodes and so are effectively unlabelled. Generally, comparing labelled networks is straightforward and can be done by comparing adjacency matrices. Unlabelled networks however, cannot easily be compared with adjacency matrices because arbitrary labelling means which nodes to compare is not clear. Similarly, any network that is not regular has a non-zero difference between itself and any of its relabellings according to an adjacency matrix despite no structural changes in the connectivity. This chapter details some possible approaches to quantify the difference between unlabelled networks by measuring distance between networks. Under this premise, networks that are similar to each other will be represented as near (small distance) each other in space and networks that are very different will be represented as far (large distance) from each other in space. This allows for a better understanding of how to search this complex space and enables the use of *point packings* to intelligently initialize optimization algorithms.

6.1   Search Space

The first issue that became apparent in the search for suitable networks was the difficulty in navigating the search space. The search space for networks of a sufficiently large size is enormous and the underlying fitness landscape is incredibly rugose. This resulted in limited ability for our algorithms to explore the search space and produce networks that were sufficiently different from the initialization. In this section, some possible representations will be examined, and their strengths and weaknesses highlighted. It is important to note

© The Author(s), under exclusive license to Springer Nature Switzerland AG 2024
J. Hughes et al., *AI Versus Epidemics*, Synthesis Lectures on Learning,
Networks, and Algorithms, https://doi.org/10.1007/978-3-031-64373-6_6

that representations are examined through the lens of the problem at hand and may benefit from revaluation for other problems. Qualities important for epidemic simulation may not be relevant for all other uses of graphs. All representations are evaluated here on undirected, unlabelled, unweighted, connected, static graphs. Because graphs are unlabelled, the nodes are not ordered according to their arbitrary labelling. Instead, they are ordered according to some property computed by the representation to avoid comparing differently labelled isomorphic graphs. The representations mentioned here do have one drawback in that it is possible to measure a distance of zero between different graphs. Technically this violates the triangle inequality property of a true distance metric, but these cases present rarely and are often not problematic as graphs that show this phenomenon are still very similar to each other. In addition, graphs that have a non-zero distance cannot be identical.

6.1.1   Numerically Representing Graphs

These different representations for network space are used along side *data driven point packing* (Stoodley et al. 2018) to find sets of sufficiently different networks for initialization. Point packing is a technique that seeks to select the maximum number of points while ensuring they are all at least some distance from each other. Therefore, the sole requirement for a point packing is a minimum distance. In the simplest cases this could be a Hamming distance (error correcting codes) or a Euclidean distance, but any distance metrics can be used. While any valid distance metric can be used, there are important implications about the representation of the problem in more complex scenarios. The distance between two points in Euclidean space is straight forward; however, the distance between networks is not so simple, especially if the networks are arbitrarily labelled. If graphs are represented in a way that permits some calculable distance between graphs, diverse collections of graphs can be packed. While simple by design, choosing a representation is complex and has large impact on outcome. There are many different options for representations and though there is likely no singular correct representation, a handful of representations are compared in the context of this problem. Different representations can be leveraged to take advantage of the positive and circumvent the negative qualities present in each. For example, inexpensive representations that trade quality for speed can be used to shoulder the computational load of early optimization so that expensive representations that trade speed for quality can be used to refine final solutions.

6.1.1.1 Diffusion Characters
Networks can be compared to each other using diffusion characters (Ashlock and Lee 2008). Diffusion characters create a square matrix of each node's pairwise connectivity by adding unique *gas* at each node and simulating diffusion. A unique gas to each node is added at the beginning of each time step and allowed to diffuse. Half of the gas is removed from each

node at the end of each time step until the system reaches equilibrium. The square matrix is collapsed into a vector by calculating column wise entropy of gases accumulating at each node. It is possible to point pack diffusion character space (R^n) using Euclidean distance on the entropy vector. Diffusion characters are expensive to compute as they require simulation. The process can be modified to improve run time by only deploying a unique gas at a subset of the nodes. This creates a partial diffusion character, trading speed for the quality of the reading.

6.1.1.2 Page Rank

Graphs can be compared to each other using Google's PageRank algorithm (Page et al. 1999). PageRank is used to rank web pages that are related to a given query. Web pages related to the query are used to assemble a network based on their linking structure (literal hyperlinks between pages). Pages are given a rank based on a value that describes the traffic received relative to the rest of the network. This differs slightly from diffusion characters in that it only measures volume of traffic through a node, not specifically where that traffic comes from. As a result, PageRank cannot distinguish between regular graphs of different degree as all nodes have the same traffic. Traffic at each node is measured relative to every other node in the network, as a result the PageRank value of a node is the proportion of the total traffic that passes throught the node. Because PageRank values are proportions, the sum of the PageRank values for all the nodes of a graph is always one. Topologically, PageRank values of a graph with n nodes lie on the $n - 1$ standard simplex. PageRank generates a vector of values in (R^n) and distance between them can be found with Euclidean Distance. PageRank is moderately expensive to compute, but it is well implemented and accessible in many popular libraries.

6.1.1.3 Degree Sequence

The degree sequence of a graph is the ordered sequence of the number of neighbours at each node (Z^n) sorted in descending order. This representation facilitates distance calculation using Hamming or Euclidean distance. The simplicity of this representation means that it is computationally very fast and inexpensive, but it may suffer from being an oversimplification as it only accounts for direct neighbors. There exist non-isomorphic graphs that have the same degree sequence and so are indistinguishable from each other through the lens of this representation.

6.1.1.4 Summary Statistics of Degree Sequence

Degree sequence gives rise to metrics based on summary statistics of degree sequence. These scale better than even the degree sequence because they do not require sorting of the sequence. In addition, while degree sequence length grows as the number of nodes in the graph increases, the summary statistics do not. They can easily be paired together to create 2 and 3 dimensional spaces that are easy to visualize. They do however suffer even more from the same oversimplification issue as different degree sequences can have the same summary statistics, meaning it may fail to identify differences between certain graph structures. This relationship is particularly interesting as mean, standard deviation, and skew are the first, second, and third moment (respectively) of the degree sequence. An important question to address is if there are any relationships between these representations and if they change depending on the size of the network.

6.1.2   Comparing Representations

In the process of determining a suitable representation for comparing graphs, many possibilities presented themselves. When similarities between the representations were discovered, it became crucial to examine and understand these similarities. One question that presented itself was if equivalencies between representations existed for all graph sizes. This experiment was created as a due diligence to establish if these relationships would hold for all graph sizes. The secondary benefit is that it also helps to quantify the strength of these relationships. The representations explored here include diffusion characters, page rank, and degree sequence. In addition, summary statistics of the degree sequence are also studied, including mean, standard deviation, and skew. Pairwise distances between the graphs are calculated using Euclidean distance.

6.1.2.1 Graph Representation Relationship Experiment

Having many possibilities for representing graphs motivates an investigation into the relationship between these different representations. One initial issue is selecting a robust way to assess these relationships. The reason this is difficult is because there is a possibility of relationships between representations changing as the size of the graphs increases. Connections between representations present on small graphs may not persist when graphs are large and vice versa. To combat this an experiment to test the relationships between representations at various graph sizes was designed. Fifty random power law cluster graphs are generated for a variety of graph sizes ranging from 5 to 325 nodes. Pairwise distances between graphs of the same size are calculated for each of the different representations. A correlation matrix is then generated of the pairwise distances of each representation, this is performed for each graph size. If representations largely agree with each other (i.e. graphs that are far apart in one representation are also far apart in the other representation), their correlation will be large. If representations have some disagreement (i.e. graphs that are far apart in one representation are close together in another representation), the correlation will be small. Linear regression is then performed for each representation comparison where the independent variable is the number of nodes, and the dependent variable is the correlation between the pairwise distances of each representation.

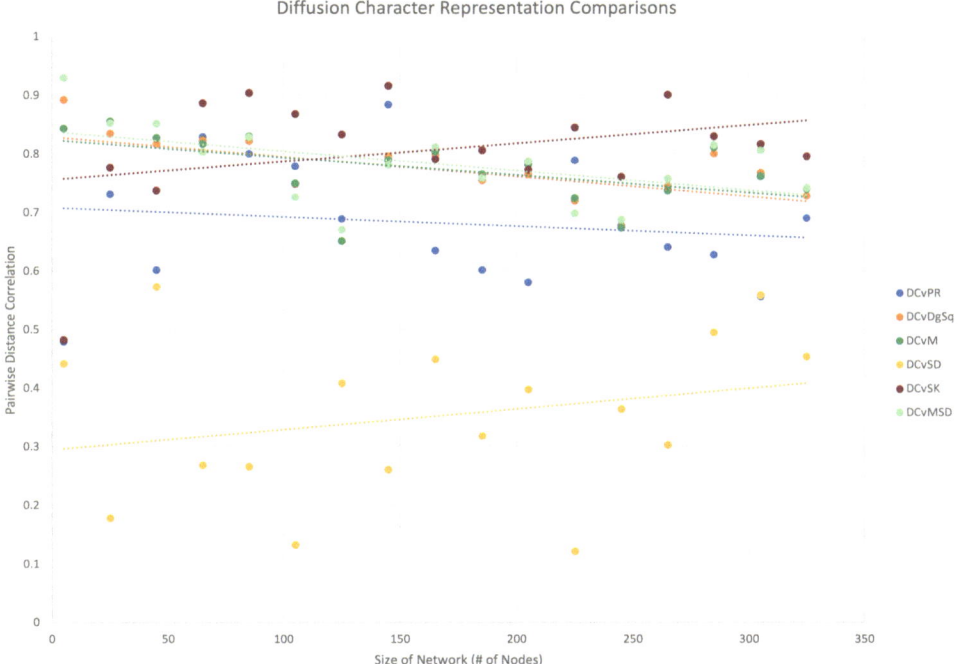

Fig. 6.1 Comparison of diffusion character graph representation with all other representations. Power law cluster graphs are generated at a variety of sizes (horizontal axis) and correlation between the pairwise distances (vertical axis) using the various representations. Linear models using parameters shown in Figs. 6.2 and 6.3 Legend codes: DC = Diffusion Characters, PR = PageRank, DeSq = Degree Sequence, M = Mean (of degree sequence), SD = Std. Deviation (of degree sequence), SK = Skew (of degree sequence), MSD = M and SD

The result is one simple linear regression line for each representation comparison. This provides an estimation of the baseline correlation (β_0) and the change in correlation as graph size increases (β_1). An example of these comparisons for diffusion characters is shown in Fig. 6.1. Each line indicates the estimation for the correlation of distances between graphs under a pair of representation. Lines that are higher up along the y-axis indicate more agreement between the pair of representations. Lines that are more horizontal indicate that the agreement between the pair of representations does not change as the size of the graph changes. Confidence intervals can be used to determine if graph size impacts the relationship between representations as well as the degree to which the representations agree with each other. Typically, when linear regression is used, slopes of zero indicate no relationship. In this case the lack of relationship means that there should be no issue using surrogate representations on larger graphs. The added benefit is that if the data can be modelled by a horizontal line, the y-intercept can be used to roughly estimate the degree to which two representations agree with one another.

β_0	Diffusion Characters	PageRank	Degree Sequence	Mean	Standard Deviation	Skew	Mean SD
Diffusion Characters		0.59281 - 0.81576	0.78348 - 0.91346	0.78262 - 0.90669	0.22023 - 0.48366	0.68738 - 0.87677	0.79187 - 0.93329
PageRank			0.54357 - 0.65465	0.42453 - 0.56133	0.14238 - 0.33394	0.60367 - 0.89704	0.49475 - 0.59919
Degree Sequence				0.87679 - 0.95563	0.3715 - 0.54793	0.65696 - 0.80855	0.95378 - 0.97908
Mean					0.15416 - 0.36539	0.52813 - 0.74674	0.92788 - 0.96685
Standard Deviation						0.08647 - 0.30264	0.43600 - 0.5961
Skew							0.55218 - 0.73884
Mean SD							

Fig. 6.2 95% confidence intervals for the y-intercept (β_0) in the linear regression exploring the relationship between graph size in nodes and correlation of pairwise distances of pairs of representations

β_1	Diffusion Characters	PageRank	Degree Sequence	Mean	Standard Deviation	Skew	Mean SD
Diffusion Characters		-0.00058 to 0.00035	**-0.00078 to -0.00023**	**-0.00073 to -0.00021**	-0.00069 to 0.00041	-0.00029 to 0.0005	**-0.00084 to -0.00024**
PageRank			-0.00044 to 0.00003	-0.00037 to 0.00021	-0.0007 to 0.00011	-0.00036 to 0.00087	**-0.00045 to -0.00001**
Degree Sequence				-0.00003 to 0.0003	-0.0003 to 0.00044	-0.00035 to 0.00029	-0.00002 to 0.00008
Mean					-0.00015 to 0.00073	-0.00018 to 0.00073	-0.00005 to 0.00012
Standard Deviation						-0.00028 to 0.00062	-0.00014 to 0.00053
Skew							-0.00021 to 0.00057
Mean SD							

Fig. 6.3 95% confidence intervals for the slope (β_1) in the linear regression exploring the relationship between graph size in nodes and correlation of pairwise distances of pairs of representations. Cells with bold values have a confidence interval that indicates the parameter estimate is significantly different from 0, indicating the relationship between representations may change as the graph size changes

The confidence intervals for β_0 give an estimate of the correlation between the two representations. It provides a measure for how similar the spaces are after projecting the graphs using the two representations. Some representations are much more highly correlated with each other. Interestingly, both more expensive representations (diffusion characters and PageRank) have simple representations that can capture very similar distances between graphs. This solidifies the possibility of using degree sequence summary statistic space in place of diffusion characters in most cases. If diffusion characters are desperately needed in some scenario, better computational time could be achieved by first optimizing with summary statistic space and only lastly corrected with diffusion characters. This would allow most of the heavy lifting to be performed by computationally inexpensive representations and refined by expensive ones. The estimates for β_0 confirm two major insights related to the relationship between expensive (diffusion characters and PageRank) and inexpensive (summary statistic) representations.

6.1.2.2 Diffusion Characters

These estimates indicate that diffusion characters are significantly less correlated to standard deviation of degree sequence than to all other metrics tested. Of the metrics that are more highly correlated with diffusion characters, there is some variability between the estimates, but no statistically significant difference. Although there is no significant difference between these levels, the highest estimate for correlation to diffusion characters is the combination of mean and standard deviation of degree sequence. While this is not significantly different from degree sequence, it provides better scaling when calculating pairwise distances as the number of dimensions is fixed and does not grow as the size of the graph grows. Additionally, two dimensions allows for intuitive visualization.

6.1.2.3 PageRank

The estimate for correlation to the PageRank metric indicate that PageRank is significantly more correlated with degree sequence and skew of degree sequence than it is to the other metrics tested. While skew is not significantly more correlated than degree sequence, the estimate is larger, and it benefits from being a single value rather than the dimension increasing with the size of the underlying network. The intervals for β_1 indicate that for the most part these relationships between representations do not change as the graph size increases. Confidence intervals that contain zero simply show zero as the estimated slope because it cannot be proven otherwise. Some intervals for the slope do not contain zero. These estimates are values with very small magnitudes and slightly negative. This indicates that the relationship may decay in graphs larger than $\sim$10,000 nodes; however, generally extrapolating that far from the sample is not advised. Small negative estimates for the slope indicate that these relationships should be reassessed if significantly larger graphs are needed but are indistinguishable from zero on the sizes of graphs discussed here.

6.1.3 Surrogate Representations

The primary reason for exploring this space is that the computational complexity of simulating an epidemic in a defined network is high. This means that optimizing for networks that facilitate types of epidemic spread is expensive because fitness updates are computationally intensive. These surrogate representations can be used to help navigate network space by suggesting graphs that are different or similar to candidate networks depending on whether exploration or exploitation is required. These tactics can offload some of the complexity of optimising networks for epidemic simulation, reducing run time and making this process significantly more feasible. Diffusion characters are expensive to calculate, but this analysis shows that a significant portion of the information that can be used to differentiate graphs with diffusion characters is preserved in some simpler metrics. While this is true, diffusion characters are still believed to offer higher quality representation because of the parallels between gas diffusion and disease spread. To circumvent the cost of computing diffusion characters, networks can be initially point packed using cheaper metrics like mean and standard deviation of degree sequence with a final pass performed using diffusion characters. Using mean and standard deviation of degree sequence as a surrogate representation for the majority of the evaluations. Of course, the degree to which each representation is used is easily changed. This allows for the best of both worlds, improved speed and confirmation of high-quality solutions.

6.2   Impact of Choice of Starting Graph

The motivation for exploring the unlabeled network search space was to investigate the underlying reason that the network optimizer is unable to find networks that are substantially different from the network it is initialized with. Analysis of the search space shows that the fitness landscape is incredible rugose. This rugosity makes it difficult to traverse through the editing commands causing exploitation to take priority over exploration, shown in Fig. 6.4. The result is a preference for finding local optima rather than a global optimum. This behaviour is particularly problematic because of the cost of explicit simulation. Because the fitness function is expensive to compute, increasing the tolerance of intermittently finding lower quality solutions to permit the discovery of new maximum fitness values become computationally prohibitive. The mix of representations presented enables navigation of the search space without epidemic simulation. These representations can be used to suggest networks that are substantially different from those already simulated, forcing the evolutionary algorithm to venture into previously unexplored areas of the search space. While this method does not guarantee the global optimum will be found, it gives higher credibility that the optimum found is a global optimum because more of the space has been searched.

Point packings are well spaced-out sets of points and have a diverse set of uses. Here, they are used to force a diverse set of networks to use for initialization, but other uses include error correction and fast clustering. Network point packings are created by adding networks to the

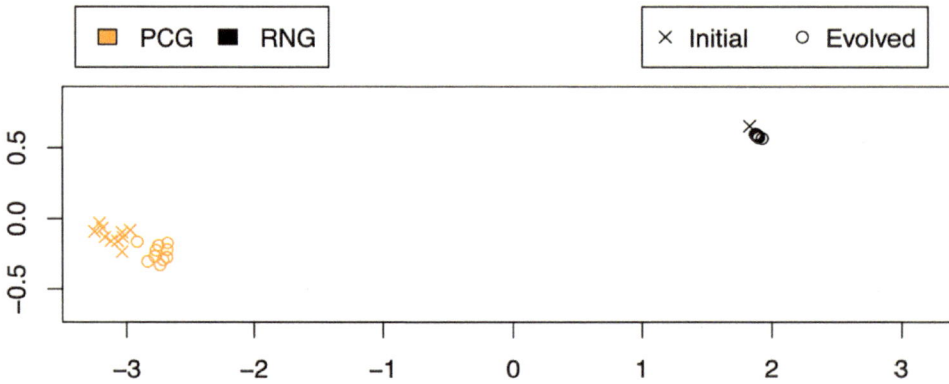

Fig. 6.4 Exploration issues in evolutionary optimization of network structure to mimic daily case numbers. Two variants of initial graphs were used: power-law cluster (yellow) and ring graphs (black). Initial graphs are shown as exes and the evolved graphs are shown as circles. These graphs are plotted on the first two principal components of their diffusion characters. Evolved graphs show little propensity to move far from their initialization. This is in line with the informal assessment that at no point in time during the optimization were drastically different solutions found

packing if they are at least some minimum distance from all other packing members. Any of the representations mentioned in the previous section are suitable, but exploiting the similarity between diffusion characters (highest quality) and summary statistic of degree sequence (computationally easiest) has proved to be very fruitful. The more distance calculations that can be performed with the given computing resources, the better and more complete the coverage of the packing will be. Complete packings enable the best initialization efficiency, maximizing the coverage of a fixed number of initialization. Point packings also require some form of random network generation to take as input. There is great flexibility in the way that networks can be generated. Generating networks throughout the search space as close to uniformly at random as possible is ideal, but not required. It is also not entirely straightforward how to accomplish such a feat and likely to be dependent on the representation that is chosen. Methods that are uniform for one representation may not be uniform in a different representation. Generating graphs for point packing can be done in many ways, but the best results were found using bit sprayers to randomly fill in adjacency matrices. Bit sprayers proved to have a significantly better coverage of the space when compared to graph generators for specific graph models such as Erdős–Rényi, Watts–Strogatz and Power-Law Cluster as is shown in Fig. 6.5.

Point packing can be performed using any graph generator, allowing for modification of the behaviour based on the type of input used. If for example, the desired graphs should be based on an existing graph model, then there is justification to use that model to generate graphs for input. However, you can also test the hypothesis that graphs of a specific model will be superior based on the probability that the optimized bit sprayer graphs could be generated under the given model. Bit sprayers have some tunable parameters that impact the bias of the resultant graph generation, but they are typically able to generate a very diverse collection of graphs. This can be seen in Fig. 6.6 along with a sample packing of graphs. The minimum distance of the packing is used to dictate the size of the packing. A smaller minimum distance allows for more graphs to be fit into the packing. The point packing works like a filter and helps to select graphs that are sufficiently different for each other to avoid redundant optimizations. The minimum distance should be tuned such that the packing roughly contains the maximum number of initializations that are feasible. Randomly selecting the same number of graphs (as the size of the packing) directly from the generator will on average involve some initializations that are very similar whereby reducing efficiency.

If one has reason to believe that a particular graph model is preferred, the appropriate generator can be used to narrow the scope of possible initializations. In the context of epidemic simulation, power-law cluster graphs are one of the graph types that can model the connectivity found in human communities and social groups well. Figure 6.7 shows the impact of initializing evolution with a point packing created using power-law cluster graphs as input. Point packed graphs result in a much greater coverage of the available area, enabling more complete search of the space. Again, it is important to note that this does not guarantee that it will outperform standard initializations on a single run, but that it

Standard deviation of degree
Mean degree

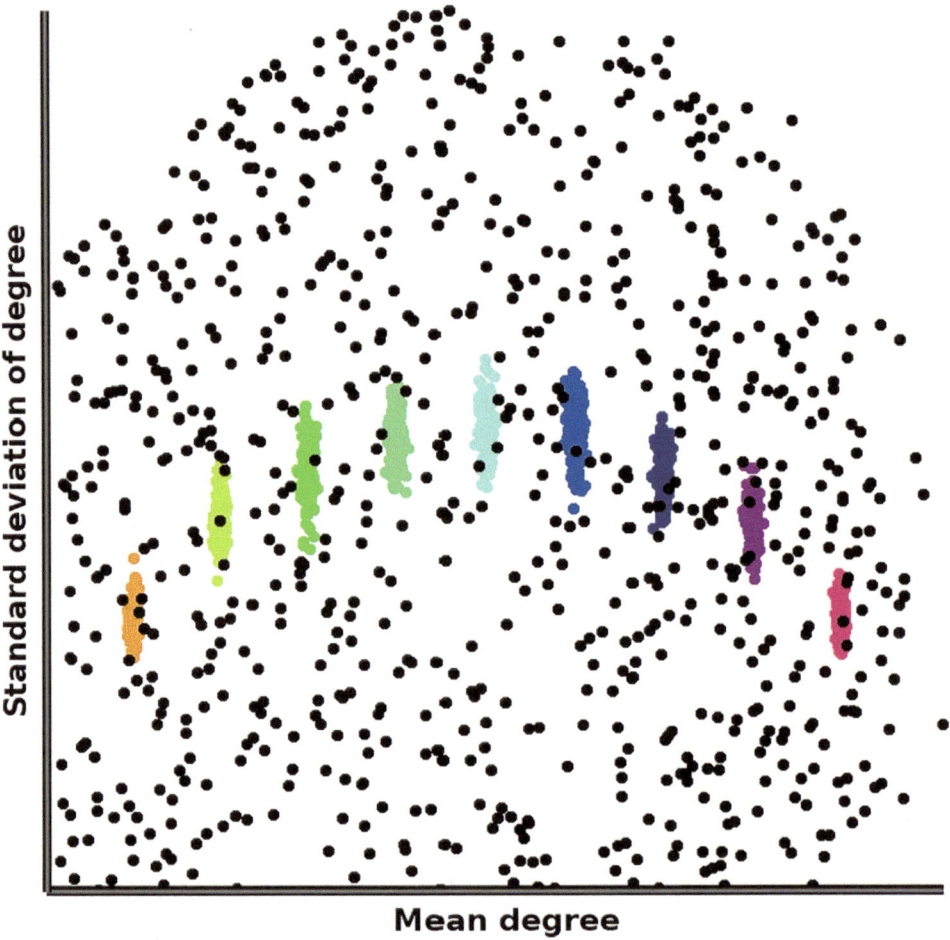

Fig. 6.5 Distribution of random graph generators using summary statistic of degree sequence as representation. Graphs generated using Bit Sprayers (Black) cover the available space much more evenly than the Erdős–Rényi graphs at variety of different parameters (various colours). Erdős–Rényi graph parameters can be modified to achieve a variety of different mean degree but tend to cluster toward central values for standard deviation of degree

will outperform it on average. Here, we can see surrogate representations in action because this point packing was performed using summary statistic of degree sequence to compute distance between networks. The separation is still present when the results are visualized with the more comprehensive and expensive diffusion characters.

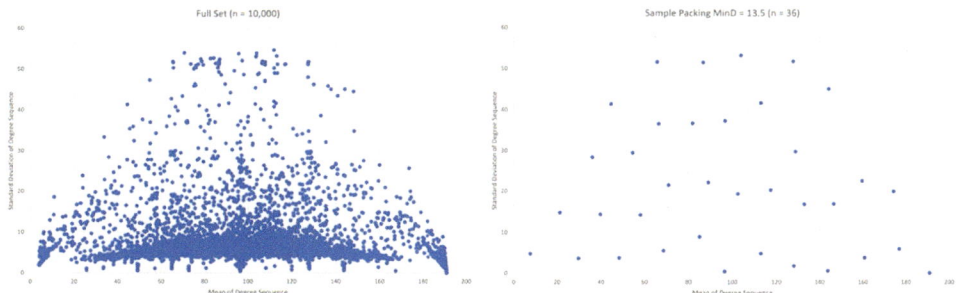

Fig. 6.6 Bit sprayer graphs and a sample point packing. Both sets shown are displayed using summary statistic of degree sequence. 10,000 graphs generated randomly using a bit sprayer (left) and a sample point packing from those graphs (right). The packing uses a minimum distance of 13.5, which results in 36 candidate graphs to be used for initialization of the network structure optimizer

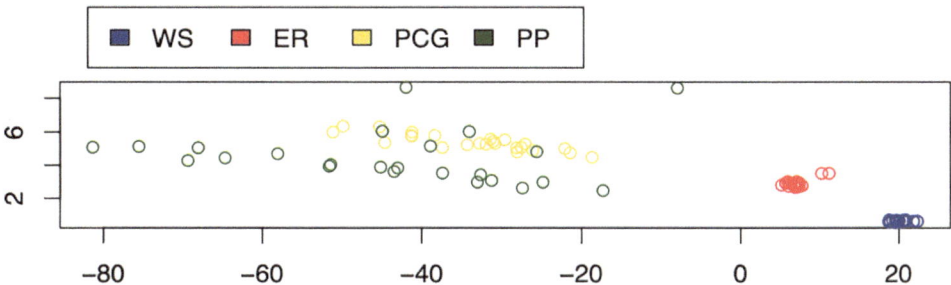

Fig. 6.7 Highest fitness networks after optimization for a disease progression profile. Networks are represented by the first two principal components of their diffusion characters. Power-law cluster (yellow), Erdős–Rényi (red) and Watts–Strogatz (blue) graphs are shown as well as a fourth initialization using a point packing with power-law cluster graphs as input (green). The point packed graphs span a significantly larger range across the space than is covered by the same number of initializations with random power-law cluster graphs. Both graphs originating from power-law cluster generation span a significantly larger area of the space than either of the other two generation methods. Interestingly all three models do occupy a unique area of the space

6.3   Impact of Choice of Patient Zero and Initiating the Epidemic

Two other components of simulating epidemic spread through a network present additional issues for accurate simulation. Both causes of these issues are centered around how the epidemic simulation begins. This section will focus on two important decisions: choosing the patient zero and when to start comparing new infections at each time step to the profile of interest. Choosing the patient zero has a different effect depending on the network, but the effect can be quite substantial. Additionally, patient zero arguably becomes a node worth labelling, which introduces the issues of considering a partially labelled network. Other problems arise from the interaction between the chosen disease model and the disease profile the network will be optimized to. Disease models with many states may contain intermediate states prior to infection to model incubation periods for a more realistic simulation. While including these features may improve the quality of the results, they can prolong the period before infection can begin to ramp appropriately. This shifts the simulated daily infection counts, prohibiting high quality matches to aggressive disease profiles. Both the issues of selecting the patient zero and accommodating models with more states will be covered here.

6.3.1   Selecting Patient Zero

Because of the stochastic nature of simulation, many replicates are required to confidently assess epidemic progression in a candidate network. The unlabeled nature of the networks introduces an additional caveat of determining where to start the epidemic. While repeated sampling can be used to get a good idea of how the epidemic will progress on average, the same approach cannot be taken to a patient zero. Randomly selecting the patient zero causes problems for the optimization of the network by convoluting the conditions under which optimization takes place. It is difficult to make alterations to the network that will constitute positive change under all possible patient zeros. Effectively, this will send mixed messages to the fitness function. Once optimization begins, the node used for patient zero should not be changed. In addition, it is not necessary randomize that part of the process.

The node labelled '0' for encoding purposes is no more suitable to be patient zero than any of the other nodes. There is both theoretical and experimental justification that all possible patient zeros must be considered. This is especially true in conjunction with a point packed initialization because the structure of the network is unique regardless of a different labelling. The disease progression starting from a node is not comparable to that found in other networks, otherwise the structure would be similar which point packing prohibits. It is possible for the choice of patient zero within a network not to have any impact on the epidemic. If the network is a regular graph, all nodes can have the same connectivity to the rest of the network. The simplest example of this is a ring graph, functionally all nodes are identical starting positions and any difference between the nodes will disappear with sufficient sampling.

To determine the extent to which the selection of patient zero impacts the spread of the epidemic through the network, an experiment was conducted comparing how the epidemic spread considering each possible patient zero in turn. Because the type of graph is expected to impact the degree to which it is important, this experiment is performed on a collection of point packed graphs to ensure a diverse set of networks is tested. The epidemic simulation is performed 100 times with each node in each network as the patient zero and the root mean squared error (RMSE) for a profile is recorded. This allows for the study of the variability of the outcomes of simulation across all possible patient zeros. The results for this experiment are shown in Fig. 6.8. While some networks are affected more than others, all networks have the capacity to change how epidemic simulation proceeds based on which patient

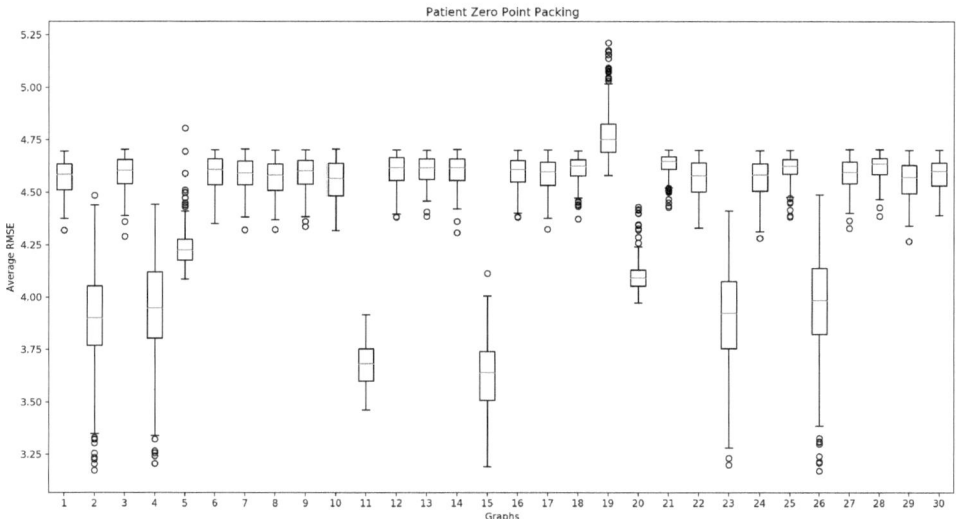

Fig. 6.8 Investigating the impact of patient zero selection. A point packing of 30 graphs each with 303 vertices are used to ensure a diverse collection of graphs are used. Graphs are point packed using summary statistic of degree sequence space. Boxplots show the distribution of the average RMSE for 100 simulations using each of the 303 vertices as patient zero. RMSE is calculated in this example to the Wellington Dufferin Guelph profile. It is important to note that all these networks are not yet optimized to fit the profile. Assessment of each patient zero will inform which node will remain patient zero during optimization

zero is chosen. Generally, the networks that have the capacity to match the profile most closely also have a large discrepancy of the epidemic progression across all possible patient zeros. Patient zero selection has the capacity to impact the progression of the epidemic and therefore, is important to consider. In addition the selection is profile specific and can be used in conjunction with the network to simulate epidemic spread matching a wide range of epidemic profiles.

Using different nodes as patient zero can have a large effect on how simulation of an epidemic proceeds through a network. The magnitude of this effect is dependent on the network and the desired disease profile. Ultimately, selecting a good patient zero will help orient the downstream optimization to the disease profile. Figure 6.9 shows more detailed information for one of the networks (network 2) from Fig. 6.8. This shows how not only are some nodes more eligible to be patient zero (for the given profile), but also that some patient zeros are subject to significantly more "randomness" with respect to the outcome of simulation. Ideally, a network will be found such that an epidemic that roughly matches the profile can be reliably simulated. Figure 6.9 shows an example of a graph that has a few very good candidate patient zero nodes (both in terms of matching and simulation consistency) for the profile in question.

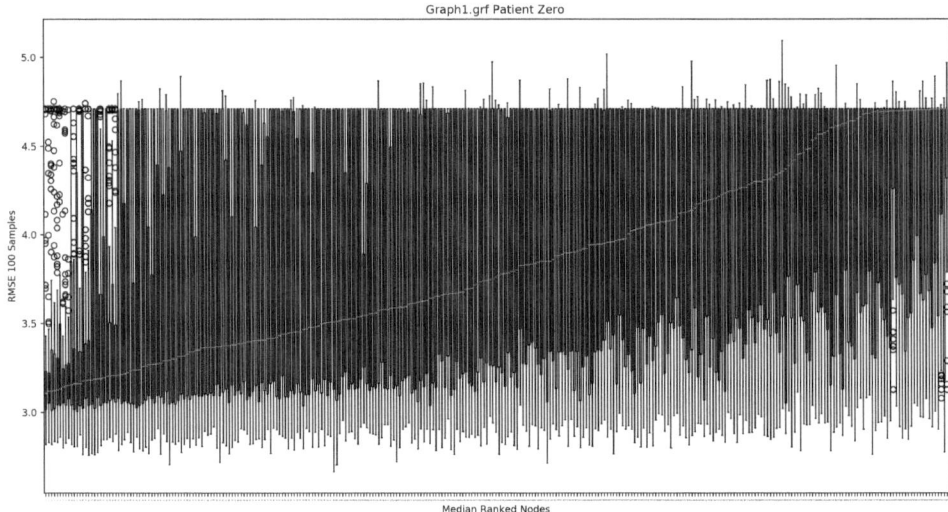

Fig. 6.9 Side-by-side box plot of RMSE from profile for 100 samples with each node as patient zero. Nodes are ordered by ascending median value. This is a more detailed view of the information that is used to create the box plot for Graph 2 in Fig. 6.5. The left most nodes are the best candidates for a patient zero that will produce a disease progression similar to the profile, whereas the right most nodes produce a disease progression that is most different from the profile. For this network and profile combination, there are wide range of outcomes depending on the patient zero that is selected. In this instance, the left most nodes also have the most consistent outcome with the least variability

6.3.2 Initiating the Epidemic

Along with selecting the patient zero there are some other issues that must be considered when initiating graph based epidemic simulation for profile matching. Two specific complications are discussed here, but there is some common ground these problems share. Both have to do with avoiding scenarios where exact matching of the profile is impossible. While it is not expected that the profile will be matched exactly, having this not be feasible indicates the possibility for undesirable bias. Two different ways this presented itself was in comparing to profiles later in the progression of the disease and when considering more complex models with additional states. Interestingly, there is one solution that addresses both issues. Both problems become trivial if the profile is matched to the best set of consecutive days, that is the set of days whose infection numbers have the lowest RMSE from the profile of choice. This solution assumes their may be some benefit to the quality of simulation if the system is allowed a period to organically enter a state from which it can accurately simulate a given profile. In addition, this approach does not punish epidemics that have very similar daily case number progression to the profile, but are offset by some number of days.

Initializing the epidemic by setting one individual's status to infected can pose a problem when matching to profiles that begin with more than one infected individual. This causes some difference from the profile to be inherently present but can also be detrimental by influencing the way the epidemic must ramp up to compensate. The result is unintentionally matching to a different profile than intended. The issue can be circumvented by either changing how the epidemic is initialized or by modifying the profile. Initializing more patient zeros is straightforward, modifying the profile is less so. If a profile represents the daily case numbers for a defined region, then it can feasibly be divided into sub-region, the sum of which would be the original profile. Profiles can be split such that all portions of the profile begin with only one infection. Both solutions do introduce additional considerations. Initializing with multiple patient zeros introduce the issue of selecting patient zeros, the number of possibilities for which grow combinatorically. Splitting the profile into separate parts can be done in many ways with no objectively correct solution. The alternative to these approaches is to initialize the epidemic with one patient zero, simulate the epidemic for a fixed number of days longer than the profile and allow profile matching to occur as a sliding window, ultimately selecting the window with the lowest RMSE to the profile. This allows for a burn-in period if required for the epidemic to ramp up at the same rate as the profile.

Accommodating models that are more complex than the Susceptible-Infected-Removed (SIR) model can help simulation more accurately reflect reality. Generally, these more complex models introduce additional states to account for exposure prior to infection as well as asymptomatic individuals. Introducing additional states, particularly between susceptible and infected states, can have some unintended consequences for the initialization of simulation; additional states cause an initial lag in cases because the minimum number of days before the first new infections are seen increases. This is of particular interest because the Susceptible-Exposed-Infected-Removed (SEIR) model is effective for simulating the spread of COVID-19 because of the addition of the exposed state to the basic SIR model. If one individual is infected on the first day (patient zero), the second day will have no new infections because individuals must pass through one or more intermediate states. The consequence is that the profile cannot possibly be matched well during the beginning of the profile and is subject to the same overcompensation discussed earlier. The issue here is that the states are empty when initialized and so are not setup organically. When an individual tests positive and is counted as a daily case, they have likely already infected other individuals (required for anything to spread). Initializing an epidemic and allowing for burn-in to occur ensures that nodes will organically be in various states when comparison to the profile begins.

To make this make this effect more extreme, the potential for a burn-in period to be useful and even necessary for more complex models with even more states. The experimental and possibly overly complicated, Susceptible-Exposed-ExposedPrime-Asymptomatic-Infected-Removed model (SEE'AIR) introduces two additional states before infection as well as the possibility for an individual to be asymptomatic, allowing them to spread the disease, but not to be counted in daily case numbers. Figure 6.10 shows the effect of allowing for a burn-in period to occur. These figures use the same set of networks, profile, and model as Figs. 6.8 and 6.9. This is a profile that has the first daily case number larger than 1 (starts after an outbreak has occurred) and uses the SEE'AIR model. The SEE'AIR model has two states

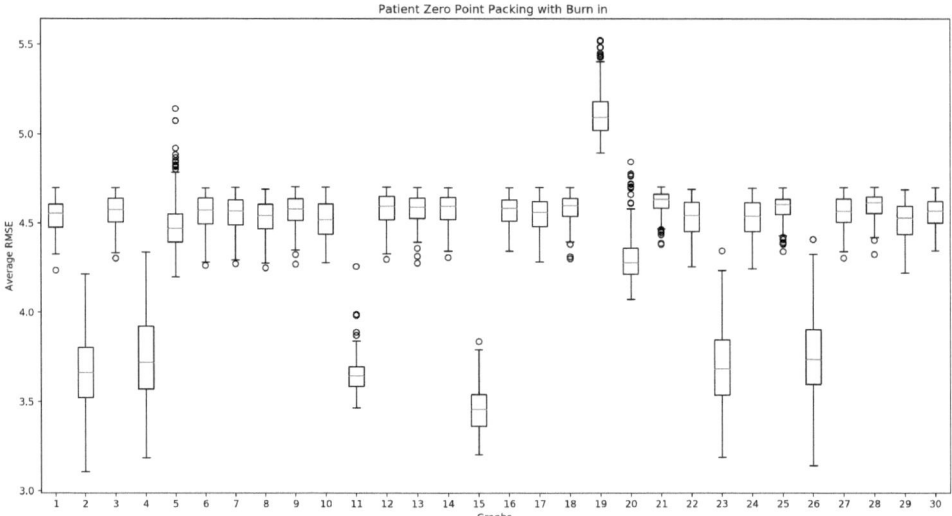

Fig. 6.10 Patient zero experiment with burn-in. This data originates from the same style of experiment that produces Figs. 6.8 and 6.9. The exception is that simulation is performed for longer, enabling a sliding window of comparison to the profile. For any single simulation this necessarily can only reduce the average RMSE, although the randomness of the 100 samples does not guarantee this outcome. This approach also seems to produce fewer outliers

that precede the infected state as well as an asymptomatic state, so it is crucial for the system to organically have nodes assigned to those states at the start of simulation. As is shown, allowing for burn in results overall in a slightly lower average RMSE and is believed to improve the generalizability of the results.

6.4   Recentering and Restarting

A notable concern with the Local THADS-N representation used in Chap. 4 to evolve personal contact networks is the fact that the final graph will at most be a distance of 256 editing commands away from the initial graph. This means that if the optimal graph exists outside this editing range, then the optimal solution can never be found. This limitation leads to many of the network induction issues detailed above. Some of these issues can be mitigated by *recentering* and *restarting* the evolutionary algorithm a number of times during evolution. After some number of generations the graph with the best fitness replaces the initial network (recentering) and evolution proceeds from the beginning using this network (restarting). Examples of the use of recentering and restarting may be found in Hughes et al. (2014a, b).

References

D. Ashlock, C. Lee, Characterization of extremal epidemic networks with diffusion characters, in *2008 IEEE Symposium on Computational Intelligence in Bioinformatics and Computational Biology* (IEEE, 2008), pp. 264–271

J.A. Hughes, S. Houghten, D. Ashlock, Recentering and restarting a genetic algorithm using a generative representation for an ordered gene problem. Int. J. Hybrid Intell. Syst. **11**(4), 257–271 (2014a)

J. Hughes, S. Houghten, G.M. Mallén-Fullerton, D. Ashlock, Recentering and restarting genetic algorithm variations for dna fragment assembly, in *2014 IEEE Conference on Computational Intelligence in Bioinformatics and Computational Biology* (2014b), pp. 1–8. https://doi.org/10.1109/CIBCB.2014.6845500

L. Page, S. Brin, R. Motwani, T. Winograd, The pagerank citation ranking: Bringing order to the web. Technical Report, Stanford InfoLab (1999)

M. Stoodley, D. Ashlock, S. Graether, Data driven point packing for fast clustering, in *2018 IEEE Conference on Computational Intelligence in Bioinformatics and Computational Biology (CIBCB)* (IEEE, 2018), pp. 1–8

Overview of Graph Theory

The algorithms that are used in this book rely on combinatorial *graphs* or *networks* used to represent the physical connections between individuals in a population. An example of a graph is displayed in Fig. A.1 in which the *nodes* represent individuals and the *edges* represent the connections between individuals. In this formulation an epidemic is able to spread from person to person through the edges. For the graph in Fig. A.1 the node with label 5 is able to infect, or be infected by, the nodes with labels 2, 3, 4, 6, 7, 8, and 52. These nodes are referred to as the *neighbours* of node 5 as they share an edge with this node, $neighbours(5) = \{2, 3, 4, 6, 7, 8, 52\}$. This section will provide a formal introduction to graph theory for those who require it.

A.1   Graph Theory

A graph G is comprised of two sets: a set of vertices (or nodes) $V(G)$ and a set of edges $E(G)$. Each edge connects exactly two vertices; the vertices connected by a given edge are said to be *incident with* that edge. A graph is stored in the computer either by using a binary adjacency matrix or using adjacency lists. For a graph with N nodes this would be realized using a NxN matrix whereby a cell of the matrix, C_{mn}, would contain a 1 if an edge exists between node m and node n and would contain a 0 if no edge exists between these nodes. Two nodes which share an edge between them are referred to as *adjacent* nodes. This would make the matrix symmetric, in other words the value of cell C_{mn} would equal C_{nm}, thus only half of the matrix is actually required to represent a network. Whereas, the adjacency list representation would be stored as N linked lists. Each list, L_i with $i \in [1, N]$, would store the nodes which are adjacent to a particular node. Therefore, list L_m would store integers representing the nodes that share an edge with node m. For example, if $L_1 = \{2, 5, 7\}$ then the node with index 1 would have an edge to nodes 2, 5, and 7. Similarly to the symmetry

J. Hughes et al., *AI Versus the Coronavirus*, Synthesis Lectures on Learning, Networks, and Algorithms, https://doi.org/10.1007/978-3-031-64373-6

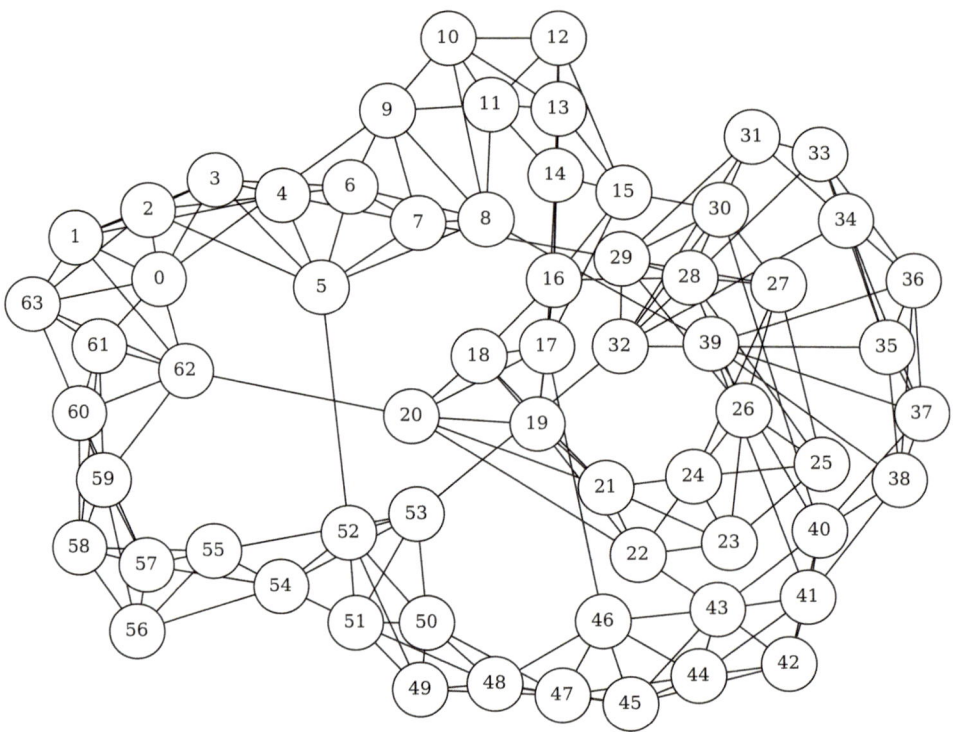

Fig. A.1 A graph with 64 nodes

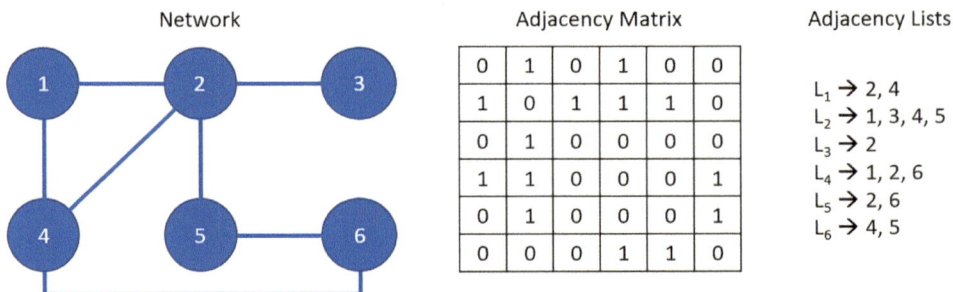

Fig. A.2 A network with six nodes and seven edges and its associated adjacency matrix and lists

seen in adjacency matrices' if $n \in L_m$ then $m \in L_n$, and vice-versa. An example network and its associated adjacency matrix and lists can be seen in Fig. A.2.

A network could be *directed* in which case an edge could exist from node m to node n without requiring an edge to exist from node n to m. This would remove the symmetric nature described in adjacency matrices and lists as outlined above. An example of a directed network and its associated adjacency matrix and lists can be seen in Fig. A.3. When con-

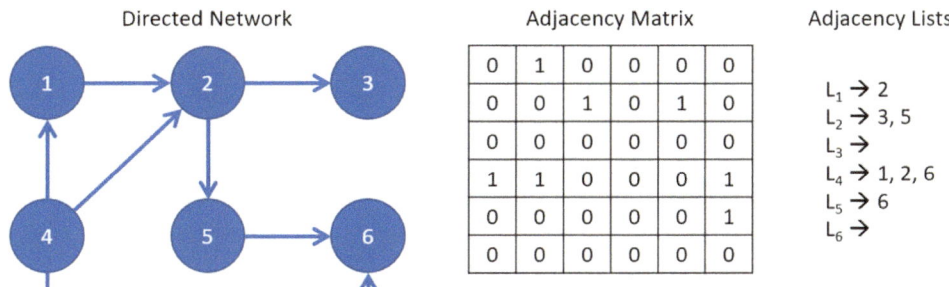

Fig. A.3 A directed network with six nodes and seven edges and its associated adjacency matrix and lists

sidering the neighbours of a node, n, using a directed graph, this concept is broken into *out-neighbours* and *in-neighbours*. Where out-neighbors are the nodes that have an edge from n to them and the in-neighbours are the nodes that have an edge from them to n. In this figure the in-neighbours of 6 are $in\text{-}neighbours(6) = \{4, 5\}$ and the out-neighbours of 4 are $out\text{-}neighbours(4) = \{1, 2, 6\}$.

Furthermore, a network could be *weighted* whereby each edge in the network is given a weight which represents the strength of that edge. When using adjacency matrices the binary restriction is removed and each cell contains a decimal or integer value which stores the strength of that particular edge or 0 meaning no edge exists. When using adjacency lists a list L_n would contain pairs of numbers (m, w) where m represents the existence of an edge from node n to node m and w stores the weight of said edge. An example of a weighted network and its associated adjacency matrix and lists can be seen in Fig. A.4.

Of course a network could be both directed and weighted by combining the two modifications described above. In this case, the adjacency matrix and lists would not be symmetric, the matrix would contain decimal or integer values or 0, and the lists would contain (node,

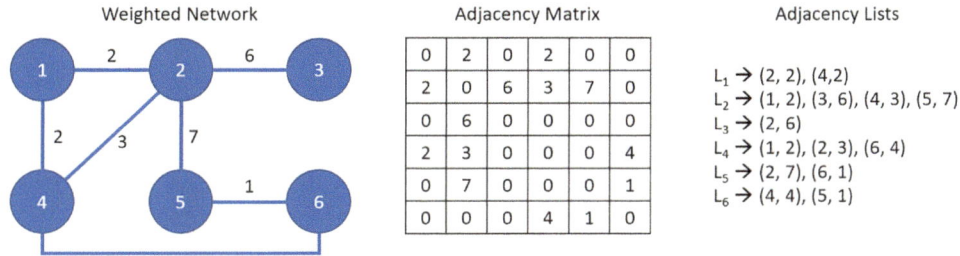

Fig. A.4 A weighted network with six nodes and seven edges and its associated adjacency matrix and lists

weight) pairs. Next some terms used to describe the attributes of a particular graph and graph centrality measures will be introduced.

The number of nodes that are connected via edges to a particular node n is known as a node's *degree*, $deg(n)$. For example in Fig. A.2 node 4 had degree $deg(4) = 3$. When a network is weighted each node, n, has two degrees: the *indegree* referring to the number of nodes with an edge from it to n ($indeg(n)$); and the *outdegree* referring to the number of nodes with an edge from n to it ($outdeg(n)$). For example in Fig. A.3 node 2 has indegree $indeg(2) = 2$ and outdegree $outdeg(2) = 2$.

A graph has a *path* from node n to m if there exists a sequence of edges that can be followed to go from n to m. If every node in the graph has a path to every other node in the graph then a graph is considered *connected*, otherwise the graph is *disconnected*. When considering directed graphs, they are *weakly connected* if it is considered connected when all the edges are replaced with undirected edges. Whereas, a directed graph is considered *strongly connected* if it features a path from any node to any other node using the directed edges. The *shortest path* between two nodes is the path between the two nodes that uses the least number of edges as part of the path. When the network is weighted, the shortest path between two nodes is the path with the lowest sum of edge weights required to connect the nodes, which isn't necessarily the least number of edges. The *distance* between two nodes is the length of the shortest path between them. The *diameter* of a network is the longest shortest path that exists for any pair of nodes in the network. Whereas, the *eccentricity* of any given node n is the largest shortest path that exists from node n to any other node in the network. Thus, the diameter of a network is equal to the maximum eccentricity of the nodes in the network.

A.2 Graph Centrality Measures

There are a number of additional features of a network, and the nodes within it, which can be used to analyse the network to determine which nodes in the network may be important when it comes to spreading a disease or vaccinating a population. Three of them used in this book are clustering coefficient, vertex cover, and shortest path frequency. These terms will be defined here.

The first centrality measure is known as the *clustering coefficient* which measures the degree to which nodes cluster together. A set of nodes are considered to cluster together based on the number of edges between said set of nodes. Consider a undirected graph with three nodes, the maximum number of edges which could exist between the nodes is three. A graph with all potential edges is referred to a *complete* graph or a *clique*, thus a graph with three nodes and three edges is a clique of size three or *triangle*. Two versions of clustering coefficients exist: *local* and *global*. The local clustering coefficient for node i, C_i, determines how close node i and it's neighbours, $neighbours(i) = N_i$, are to forming a clique. The local clustering coefficient for undirected graphs can be calculated using Eq. A.1 below. The notation e_{jk} refers to an edge from node j to node k and the vertical lines around a set, $|\{...\}|$, returns the number of items contained within the set. A value of $C_i = 1$ indicates that the nodes i and those in it's neighbourhood form a complete graph (clique) as all potential edges are present.

$$C_i = 2\frac{|\{e_{jk} : j, k \in N_i, e_{jk} \in E\}|}{deg(i)(deg(i) - 1)} \tag{A.1}$$

When considering directed graphs Eq. A.1 is modified by removing the factor of 2, resulting in Eq. A.2:

$$C_i = \frac{|\{e_{jk} : j, k \in N_i, e_{jk} \in E\}|}{deg(i)(deg(i) - 1)} \tag{A.2}$$

Furthermore, the global clustering coefficient is a measure of the number of triangles that exists compared to the number of triangles possible in the network. This is calculated using *triplets*, which is a set of three nodes that are connected by two (*open triplet*) or three edges (*closed triplet*). Therefore, the global clustering coefficient is also a measure of the number of closed triplets compared to the number of closed and open triplets in the network. The number of closed triplets can be calculated using an adjacency matrix A: $\sum_{i,j,k} A_{ij} A_{jk} A_{ki}$. And the number of open and closed triplets can be calculated as follows: $\sum_i deg(i)(deg(i) - 1)$. Together this results in Eq. A.3 for calculating the global clustering coefficient for a network.

$$C = \frac{\sum_{i,j,k} A_{ij} A_{jk} A_{ki}}{\sum_i deg(i)(deg(i) - 1)} \tag{A.3}$$

The second centrality measure is known as the *minimal vertex cover* and it provides the smallest set of nodes from a network, $S \subset V$, such that every edge in the network E has at least one endpoint in the set S. This measure is useful when determining which nodes in the network are well-connected and/or required in order to connect to the nodes on the periphery of the network. Thus, this can be used to determine which nodes to vaccinate when determining the optimal vaccination strategy.

The final centrality measure is *shortest path frequency* and it measures the number of shortest paths that any given node of the network is contained within. First, the shortest paths between any pair of nodes are determined. Then, the number of said paths that contain a particular node, n, is returned as the shortest path frequency for that node. Nodes that are contained in several shortest paths are likely to be important for the disease to propagate across the network, hence they are also important to be chosen for vaccination.